CLINICAL BIOCHEMISTRY

2nd edition

R. Luxton

Senior Lecturer in Clinical Chemistry, Department of Biological and Biomedical Sciences, University of the West of England, Bristol, UK

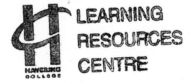

Scion

Second edition © Scion Publishing Ltd, 2008

ISBN 978 1904842 41 5

First edition published in 1999 by Butterworth-Heinemann (ISBN 0 7506 2878 2)

A CIP catalogue record for this book is available from the British Library.

Scion Publishing Limited
Bloxham Mill, Barford Road, Bloxham, Oxfordshire OX15 4FF
www.scionpublishing.com

Important Note from the Publisher

Typeset by Phoenix Photosetting, Chatham, Kent, UK
Printed by Gutenberg Press, Malta

Contents

Processing

Preface

This second edition maintains the ethos of the first edition in being designed and written for the student who has no previous experience or knowledge of clinical biochemistry. It covers the breadth of the topic, presenting the essential facts needed to understand the role of clinical biochemistry laboratories in the investigation of disease and how these investigations are performed. The different subject areas are presented in a simple manner, giving definitions and explanations of the essential principles of clinical biochemistry. This is not intended to be an in-depth text and therefore some of the more specialized investigations are not covered or are only mentioned in passing. The second edition introduces some of the newer technologies being used in biomedical science for understanding and diagnosing disease. These include lateral flow immunoassays, two-dimensional electrophoresis, biosensors and the use of receiver-operator-characteristic curves to evaluate diagnostic tests. In addition, the references given with each chapter have been revised and updated.

Each chapter begins with a set of learning objectives for students. After studying the chapter they should be able to complete the learning objectives. The chapter gives a brief introduction to the topic, followed by a discussion on the pathophysiology and role of the clinical biochemistry department in the investigation of some of the more relevant diseases. There is a brief review of methodology used in particular investigations and some chapters give a more detailed description of the more generic techniques. At the end of the chapter is a reading list pointing to other books and review papers that give a more detailed and applied discussion on particular aspects of each topic. Self-assessment questions allow readers to check they have understood the essential facts and concepts in the chapter. The questions address the learning objectives set out at the beginning of the chapter, and answers are given at the end of the book. Side boxes in the chapters give historical background to some of the topics, worked examples of important calculations and some interesting facts.

This book's novel organizational design is based on a systems analysis type approach, where the body functions are divided into six main areas. The areas are; input, control, processing, transport and storage, defence and output. In each of these sections a number of topics are presented in a manner to show the role of the clinical biochemistry laboratory in the investigation of diseases related to that topic.

Chapters 2 and 3 cover input: the topics relating to nutrition and digestion. The section on control, Chapters 4–9, covers the principle of genetic control and its loss, and aspects of endocrinology (chemical control). This is not a comprehensive review of all aspects of endocrinology but an overview introducing the more important hormonal systems and concepts encountered in most clinical biochemistry laboratories. Chapters 10 and 11 cover processing, which studies how enzymes are used in the investigation of disease; in particular, diseases causing cell damage and diseases involving mutated enzymes. Aspects of transport and storage are covered in Chapters 12–14 and include diseases associated with plasma proteins, lipids, acid balance and blood gases. An area that is sometimes overlooked is the defence systems of the body, which are covered in Chapters 15 and 16. In these two chapters the role of the clinical biochemistry laboratory in the investigation of diseases associated with the immune system is covered. There may be a certain amount of overlap with some immunology departments but the material in this text does reflect the biochemical aspects of these investigations. Finally, and logically, is the output of waste, covered in Chapters 17 and 18. These final two chapters concentrate on the biochemical investigation of renal and liver disease.

I believe this text gives a sufficiently broad introduction to the subject of clinical biochemistry so that the student will have the necessary basic understanding and knowledge to appreciate the role of the clinical biochemistry laboratory in the investigation of disease. This includes not only the range of investigations undertaken, but also how various parameters are measured. This text will also give the student sufficient grounding in the subject to allow further in-depth study of the various topics covered.

R. Luxton
January 2008

Abbreviations

1,25-DHCC	1,25-dihydroxycholecalciferol
25-HCC	25-hydroxycholecalciferol
AAS	atomic absorption spectrophotometry
ACTH	adrenocorticotropic hormone
ADH	antidiuretic hormone
ALT	alanine aminotransferase
AST	aspartate aminotransferase
AVP	arginine vasopressin
BMR	basal metabolic rate
CA	carbohydrate antigen
CCK-PZ	cholecystokinin-pancreozymin
CFTR	cystic fibrosis transmembrane conductance regulator
CK	creatine kinase
CRH	corticotrophin-releasing hormone
CV	coefficient of variation
DELFIA	dissociation-enhanced lanthanide fluorescence immunoassay
DNA	deoxyribonucleic acid
ECF	extracellular fluid
ELISA	enzyme-linked immunosorbent assay
EMIT	enzyme-multiplied immunoassay technique
FSH	follicle-stimulating hormone
FTI	free thyroxine index
GFR	glomerular filtration rate
GGT	γ-glutamyltransferase
GH	growth hormone
GIP	gastric inhibitory polypeptide
GLC	gas–liquid chromatography
GRH	growth hormone-releasing hormone
Hb	haemoglobin
HDL	high-density lipoprotein
HPA	hypothalamic–pituitary axis
HPLC	high-performance liquid chromatography
HPTA	hypothalamine–pituitary–thyroid axis
IBEM	inborn error of metabolism
ICF	intracellular fluid
IDDM	insulin-dependent diabetes mellitus
IDL	intermediate-density lipoprotein
IFN	interferon

IRMA	immunoradiometric assay
ISE	ion-selective electrode
JGA	juxtaglomerular apparatus
LDH	lactate dehydrogenase
LDL	low-density lipoprotein
LH	luteinizing hormone
MAC	membrane attack complex
MEC	minimum effective concentration
mRNA	messenger ribonucleic acid
MTC	minimum toxic concentration
NIDDM	non-insulin-dependent diabetes mellitus
PCR	polymerase chain reaction
pI	isoelectric point
PKU	phenylketonuria
PRL	prolactin
PSA	prostate-specific antigen
PTH	parathyroid hormone
PTHrp	parathyroid hormone-related peptide
QC	quality control
RDA	recommended daily allowance
RIA	radioimmunoassay
ROC	receiver-operator-characteristic
SIADH	syndrome of inappropriate antidiuresis
SRBC	sheep red blood cells
T_3	triiodothyronine
T_4	thyroxine
TBG	thyroxine-binding globulin
TLC	thin-layer chromatography
TRH	thyrotrophin-releasing hormone
tRNA	transfer ribonucleic acid
TSH	thyroid-stimulating hormone
UDPGT	uridyl diphosphate glucuronosyl transferase
VIP	vasoactive intestinal polypeptide
VLDL	very-low-density lipoprotein

What is clinical biochemistry?

Learning objectives

After studying this chapter you should confidently be able to:

- **Give an overview of the role of a clinical biochemistry laboratory.**
  To aid in the diagnosis, screening, prognosis and monitoring of disease by the analysis of biological fluids. Blood is the most common sample sent to the laboratory; plasma is obtained from an anticoagulated blood sample, and serum is obtained from a clotted blood sample.

- **Describe the variables affecting a biochemical test.**
  Analytical factors that affect a result are imprecision, accuracy, sensitivity and specificity – physiological factors include: gender, age, race, diet, stress, posture and diurnal rhythm.

- **Define the meaning of reference ranges and measures of clinical utility.**
  Reference ranges are usually constructed by studying a healthy population. The clinical utility of a test is a measure of how well a biochemical test can discriminate between healthy and disease groups of patients. Clinical sensitivity is the proportion of positive test results in a disease population expressed as a percentage, and clinical specificity is the proportion of negative results in a healthy population expressed as a percentage. A ROC curve allows the utility of different tests to be compared.

- **Describe the units of measurement used in clinical biochemistry laboratories.**
  The most common unit of measurement is mmol/l and enzyme activity is usually measured in iu/l.

The human being is a highly complex collection of cells organized into the tissues and organs that we call our body. Every living cell in our body, whether it is a free-floating blood cell or a muscle cell in the leg, contains a huge array of different chemicals all interacting and reacting in highly organized and predetermined ways. These are the chemical reactions of life, the biochemistry of the cell. The structured chemical reactions taking place every second throughout the life of the cell form the metabolic pathways studied by biochemists.

Every living organism and cell must be able to perform a number of functions to remain healthy. These are to:

- **Input** energy and basic building material for growth and sustenance;
- Respond to **control** mechanisms, which direct and co-ordinate its functions;
- **Process** the building material to make required products for export, growth and division;
- **Transport and store** ingested (input) building material or synthesized product;
- **Defend** itself against pathogens;
- **Output** or remove toxic and waste products.

If any of the above functions fail, the body or cell will become sick, which we recognize as disease.

This book is divided into six sections; **Input**, **Control**, **Processing**, **Transport and Storage**, **Defence** and **Output**. Each section contains chapters related to aspects of clinical biochemistry based on that basic biochemical function, the pathology that can result when there is a breakdown in the process and the biochemical investigation of that breakdown. Case studies highlight the important concepts in the chapter and boxes point the reader to related topics and case studies in other chapters.

1.1 THE ROLE OF THE CLINICAL BIOCHEMISTRY LABORATORY

In health, we are unaware of the hundreds of thousands of biochemical reactions maintaining and sustaining our bodies. When the chemistry of the cell is altered, or one of the controlling signals becomes defective, the normal metabolic process breaks down, causing unusual chemicals and abnormal amounts of everyday chemicals to be synthesized, which find their way out of the cell and into the blood. The change in the metabolic process can often manifest itself as a disease.

The clinical biochemistry laboratory analyses blood samples and other body fluids such as urine, to detect and measure a range of different chemicals in the sample (see *Box 1.1*). The clinician looking after the patient sends the samples to the laboratory to:

- Help make a diagnosis;
- Confirm a diagnosis;
- Screen for latent disease;
- Help to evaluate the prognosis;
- Monitor disease progress.

In the following chapters you will see how these different roles apply to different tests performed on biochemical samples (see *Box 1.2*).

The laboratory receives the sample, performs the analysis and sends the result of the test to the requesting physician. Computers in the laboratory enable the doctor to access patients' results simply and quickly from a

> **Box 1.1 Types of sample analysed in a clinical biochemistry laboratory**
>
> ■ Blood, plasma and serum
> ■ Urine
> ■ Cerebrospinal fluid
> ■ Synovial fluid
> ■ Gastric fluid
> ■ Duodenal fluid
> ■ Synovial fluid
> ■ Tears
> ■ Saliva

> **Box 1.2 One of the earliest recorded diagnostic tests on a body fluid was for diabetes.**
>
> Approximately 1500 years ago the Chinese doctor Chen Ch'uan was testing urine for 'sweetness', from the glucose present, to detect diabetes. It was not until the beginning of the 20th century that diseases were diagnosed by composition of body fluids, and Sir Archibald Garrod was able to demonstrate that patients with alcaptonuria produced urine that turned black on standing.
>
> In the 1940s and 1950s the development of instrumental techniques such as spectroscopy and chromatography were applied to the chemical analysis of human material and developed into the subject of clinical biochemistry as we know it today. In the 1970s and 1980s, we saw a revolution in the degree of automation and range of tests available, allowing a rapid turnaround of result for the clinician. The 1990s saw the emergence of molecular biology and its application to the monitoring, screening and diagnosis of diseases such as cancer.

remote terminal, and direct requesting of tests is also possible. Storage of patients' results allows previous tests performed to be inspected with the current result, thereby allowing changes over many days, weeks or months to be monitored.

1.2 WHAT DOES THE RESULT MEAN?

Once an analysis has been performed on a sample sent to the clinical biochemistry laboratory, the result sent back to the clinician has to be interpreted: what does it mean? To be of use to the clinician a number of factors need to be known about the test before it can be useful; for example, knowing the concentration of potassium in a blood sample is useless unless you also know what concentration is found in a healthy person. Two types of factor can be considered: analytical factors and physiological factors.

Analytical factors affecting a result

Various analytical factors can affect a result. These are: imprecision, accuracy, sensitivity and specificity.

For a biochemical measurement to be useful, it is important to know about the method used to measure that **analyte** (the substance or compound being measured). Two important features of a method are its imprecision and accuracy. These are monitored day to day by the laboratory and have to be kept within well-defined limits. The sensitivity and specificity of the method are also important, and these are defined when the method is first developed.

The term **imprecision** indicates how close the results from repeated measurements of the same sample lie (see *Fig. 1.1*). The **coefficient of variation** (CV) is often used as a measure of the imprecision and is often expressed as a percentage:

$$\text{Coefficient of variation} = \frac{\text{standard deviation of repeated measurements}}{\text{mean value of repeated measurements}} \times 100$$

The term **accuracy** defines how close a result is to the true answer. Accuracy can be assessed using reference material with known values for the test of interest. The percentage deviation from the true result for the working or routine method can be then calculated.

The term **sensitivity** is often used to define the detection limit of a method, that is, the lowest concentration of analyte that can be measured and distinguished from zero concentration.

The term **specificity** is an indication of the extent to which other chemicals in the sample interfere in the measurement of an analyte by a given method. A specific method is one that only measures the analyte of interest, whereas in a non-specific method many other substances may react, giving a falsely elevated result. It is therefore important to know what substances in the sample besides the analyte will also be measured by a given method.

The analytical performance of a method is monitored day to day using quality control (QC) samples with known concentrations of analyte. The QC samples are measured several times a day and the variations in the results reflect the imprecision, and differences from the true value indicate accuracy.

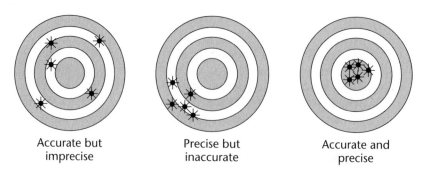

Accurate but   Precise but   Accurate and
imprecise   inaccurate   precise

Figure 1.1
Target showing the effect of accuracy and imprecision.

Physiological factors affecting a result

Every individual has their own biochemical reactions taking place in their cells under the control of their own hormones and enzymes, resulting in an individual biochemical profile. The biochemical profile is the different concentrations of a selection of analytes measured in blood samples from that individual. Every individual will have a slightly different biochemical profile due to genetic and other differences such as age, gender and race – this is **inter-individual variation**.

In addition, there are other factors that can affect our own, particular biochemical profile day to day. We can often influence and modify these factors which include: diet, stress, posture, time of the month (some hormones have monthly cycles), time of day (some hormones have daily cycles or a **diurnal rhythm**), level of fitness and geographical location. These factors contribute to **intra-individual variation**.

When a result is interpreted, the above factors that can influence the concentration of a particular analyte in the absence of a pathological process must be considered, otherwise a false conclusion may be drawn.

1.3 REFERENCE RANGES

As an aid to interpretation, a result from a clinical laboratory is compared with a **reference range**. For each analyte the reference range is calculated using results from a group of healthy volunteers called the **reference population**. This used to be called the normal range and normal population, but due to difficulties in defining 'normal', the term 'reference' is preferred. Some analytes are affected by inter-individual variables such as age or gender, and reference ranges have to reflect these differences. To do this the reference population has to be selected carefully to include only individuals of a certain gender or age range. Thus for a particular analyte there may be a number of reference ranges that reflect different age groups or gender. In the interpretation of a result, the reference range used will depend on the gender or age of the patient being investigated.

The reference range is calculated to include 95% of the test values from the reference population, the top and bottom 2.5% being excluded. This will mean that a healthy person will have a one in 20 chance that their result will fall outside the reference range. Where the analyte has a **normal** distribution, the reference range can be taken to be the average or **mean** value plus and minus 2 standard deviations, as shown in *Fig. 1.2*. In some instances the reference population has a skewed distribution which can be 'normalized' by using the log value of the analyte concentration: this is called a **log normal** distribution.

1.4 CLINICAL UTILITY

When a biochemical measurement is used to detect latent or preclinical disease it must be able to differentiate between patients with the disease

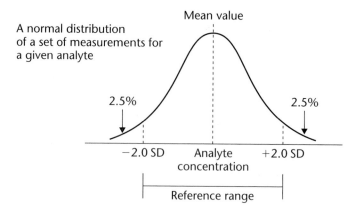

Figure 1.2
Normal distribution of a set of measurements for a given analyte, showing the reference range, which includes values plus or minus two standard deviations (SD) from the mean value.

and healthy patients. This is of particular importance when using the biochemical test as a screening test, for example, a pregnancy test or a test for prostate cancer. We have already seen that for a given group of patients there will be a spread of results for a given biochemical test. For healthy people this gives rise to the reference range shown in *Fig. 1.2*. To be useful, the result from a patient with a disease should lie outside the reference range. Taking many results from patients with that disease will give a range of values for that biochemical test. Ideally there will be no overlap between the two frequency distributions of results from the healthy and disease patients (see *Fig. 1.3a*). More often than not, the ideal situation is not achieved and there is an overlap between the two sets of results, as shown in *Fig. 1.3b*. This leads to a grey area in which the result could have come from a healthy patient or one with the disease. In this situation a cut-off value is chosen, above which the result is said to belong to the disease group and below which the result belongs to the healthy group. By introducing the cut-off value there will be some results placed into the wrong group. Results from the healthy population above the cut-off value will be **false positives** and results from the disease population falling below the cut-off value will be **false negatives**.

The usefulness of a biochemical test in detecting disease is evaluated by two measures of clinical utility; these are **clinical sensitivity** and **clinical specificity**. Do not confuse these terms with analytical sensitivity and specificity, which were discussed earlier in the chapter.

Clinical sensitivity can be defined as the proportion of positive test results in the disease group expressed as a percentage, given by the following equation:

$$\text{Sensitivity} = \frac{\text{TP}}{\text{TP} + \text{FN}} \times 100$$

(a)

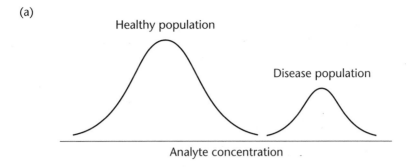

(b)

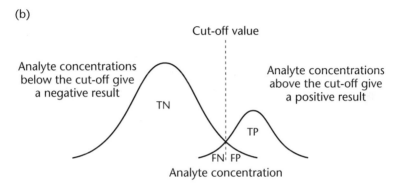

Figure 1.3
(a) Two hypothetical populations showing no overlap between healthy and disease patients for a given analyte. A more realistic situation is shown in (b) where the test result can classify the patients according to whether they have a positive or negative test and by the population they are from. Four groups are recognized; true negatives (TN) – healthy subjects with a negative test; true positives (TP) – disease subjects with a positive test; false negatives (FN) – disease subjects with a negative result; false positives (FP) – healthy subjects with a positive test.

where TP is the number of true positive results and FN is the number of false negative results.

Clinical specificity can be defined as the proportion of negative test results in the healthy group expressed as a percentage, given by the following equation:

$$\text{Specificity} = \frac{\text{TN}}{\text{TN} + \text{FP}} \times 100$$

where TN is the number of true negative results and FP is the number of false positive results.

An ideal test where there is no overlap of test results from the disease and healthy groups will have a sensitivity and specificity of 100%. See *Box 1.3* for an example.

The calculated sensitivity and specificity of a test depends on the **cut-off value** chosen to differentiate between the healthy and disease groups. If the cut-off value is lowered then there will be fewer false negatives, so the

---

Box 1.3 A new test for the detection of bowel cancer has been developed and is now being evaluated for clinical use.

One hundred healthy volunteers and 100 patients with bowel cancer were all screened using the new diagnostic test. Initial studies were undertaken to determine the concentration at which to place a cut-off level. A result greater than the cut-off level is considered to be a positive result, indicating the presence of bowel cancer. A result less than the cut-off level is considered a negative result. In the healthy group, four subjects gave a positive test. From the group of patients with bowel cancer, 92 gave a positive test. From these data the clinical utility of the new test can be determined. In a perfect situation none of the healthy group should give a positive result and none of the disease group should give a negative result. From this study the following were found:

$$\text{Sensitivity} = \frac{92}{92 + 8} \times 100 = 92\%$$

$$\text{Specificity} = \frac{96}{96 + 4} \times 100 = 96\%$$

In other words, this means that the new screening test for bowel cancer will be positive in 92% of those patients with the disease and, at the same time, negative in 96% of healthy people. This implies that 4% of healthy people who have the test will be told they have cancer when in fact they do not. On the other hand, the test will miss 8% of patients with cancer.

---

sensitivity of the test increases, but there will be more false positives, thereby reducing the specificity. The converse is also true, that by increasing the cut-off value there will be fewer false positives (greater specificity) but more false negatives (reduced sensitivity). This shows that there is an optimum cut-off value to be chosen which maximizes both sensitivity and specificity.

Other useful measures of clinical utility are the predictive values, the **positive predictive value** and the **negative predictive value**. These values give the probability that the result will correctly categorize the patient. The positive predictive value is the probability that a patient giving a positive result will be a member of the disease population and is given by the following equation:

$$\text{Positive predictive value} = \frac{TP}{TP + FP} \times 100$$

The negative predictive value is the probability of a negative result arising from a healthy individual and is given by the following equation:

$$\text{Negative predictive value} = \frac{TN}{TN + FN} \times 100$$

Ideally, the predictive values should be 100%, which is found when there is no overlap between the results of the test performed on healthy and disease populations. The predictive values are useful to the clinician as they give the probability of the patient actually having, or not having the disease.

The above measures of clinical utility are defined for a given cut-off value but another technique has been used to assess the overall performance of the test using the sensitivity and specificity calculated at different cut-off values: this is called the **receiver–operator–characteristic (ROC) curve**. In this technique the sensitivity and 1 − specificity are plotted for different cut-off values, starting at low test concentrations (100% sensitivity), increasing in value to high test concentrations (100% specificity). In a perfect test where there is no overlap in test results between the healthy (or control) population and the disease population, the ROC curve will be a right-angled line that goes from 0,0 to 0,100 and then to 100,100 on the graph. With increasing degrees of overlap between the healthy and disease population, the line on the ROC curve moves further from the top left-hand corner of the graph (0,100). *Figure 1.4* shows a typical ROC curve. The advantage of the ROC curve is that different tests can be compared with each other. The test that gives a line closest to the top left-hand corner of the graph is the test with the best overall performance. There are a number of different methods used to calculate which ROC curve is the best; for example, by measuring the area under the curve (see *Box 1.4*).

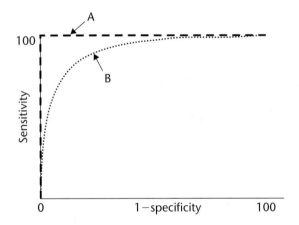

Figure 1.4
Line A is a ROC curve obtained when there is no overlap between healthy and disease populations. Line B is the ROC curve when there is a degree of overlap between the healthy and disease populations.

Box 1.4 ROC curves

ROC curves were first used to analyse radar signals in the Second World War as a way of correctly identifying aircraft from the incoming signals. Later, in the 1950s, ROC curves were used in psychophysics research to assess the ability of humans to perceive 'weak signals'. The point of using ROC curves in all these applications is to reduce the numbers of false positives and false negatives.

1.5 BLOOD SAMPLES

The majority of tests are performed on blood samples. They are taken from the patient into special bottles that often contain an **anticoagulant** to prevent the blood from clotting. The majority of biochemical measurements are performed on plasma or serum (see *Fig. 1.5*). Plasma is the clear fluid from an anticoagulated blood sample and contains fibrinogen. Serum is the clear fluid from a blood sample that has been placed into a plain sterile tube and allowed to clot, so will not contain fibrinogen.

The most commonly used anticoagulants used include:

- Lithium heparin;
- Fluoride/oxalate;
- EDTA.

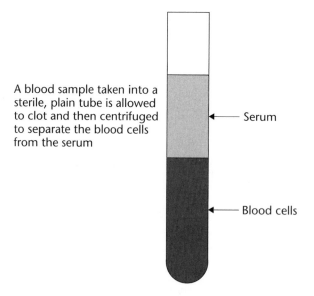

A blood sample taken into a sterile, plain tube is allowed to clot and then centrifuged to separate the blood cells from the serum

← Serum

← Blood cells

Figure 1.5
Diagram of separated blood in a sample tube.

1.6 UNITS OF MEASUREMENT

By convention the units used within a clinical biochemistry laboratory are based on the *Système International d'Unités*, the SI system of measurement. The basic physical measurements, units and symbols are:

- Length – metre (m);
- Mass – kilogram (kg);
- Time – second (s).

Under this system volumes are defined as a cubic quantity of length, for example m^3, cm^3. In practice, the metric system is still widely used in clini-

Table 1.1 Decimal multiples and submultiples used with SI and metric units

Multiple	Prefix	Symbol	Submultiple	Prefix	Symbol
10	deca	da	10^{-1}	deci	d
10^3	kilo	k	10^{-2}	centi	c
10^6	mega	M	10^{-3}	milli	m
10^9	giga	G	10^{-6}	micro	μ
10^{12}	tera	T	10^{-9}	nano	n
10^{15}	peta	P	10^{-12}	pico	p
10^{18}	exa	E	10^{-15}	femto	f
			10^{-18}	atto	a
			10^{-21}	zepto	z

cal laboratories and in medical practice, where the unit of volume is the litre (rather than the SI unit dm^3). For larger or smaller numbers of units, that is, more than a thousand or less than a thousandth, there are a number of multiples and submultiples that are used in conjunction with the unit names, as shown in *Table 1.1*.

Small volumes are often measured in millilitres (ml) which are equivalent to the SI unit cm^3, and even smaller volumes are measured in microlitres (μl). It is important to understand the relationship between the prefixes used in the units of measurement.

For example:

■ There are **1000 μl in 1 ml** (1 cm^3);
■ There are **1000 ml in 1 litre** (1 dm^3).

Most measurements made in the clinical biochemistry laboratory are in concentration units. This is the amount of a substance present in a given volume, for example, the number of grams in a litre or milligrams in a millilitre. The SI name for the unit of concentration is the **mole**, where **1 mole is the formula weight of that substance, measured in grams, dissolved in 1 litre of solvent (usually water).**

A 1 molar solution is equivalent to 1 mol/l and is written as a 1 M solution, i.e.

$$1 \text{ mol l}^{-1} = 1 \text{ M}$$

Most physiological measurements are 1000 or more times less concentrated than molar units, so the common concentration units used in the clinical biochemistry laboratory are:

mmol l^{-1} – formula weight in milligrams dissolved in 1 litre
$\mu\text{mol l}^{-1}$ – formula weight in micrograms dissolved in 1 litre
nmol l^{-1} – formula weight in nanograms dissolved in 1 litre

For some hormones, which are present in extremely low concentrations, pmol l^{-1} or even fmol l^{-1} are used.

For substances where it is difficult to obtain an accurate formula weight, concentration units are given by the weight of compound in a given volume of solvent. **Proteins** are measured in this manner; for example, it is common to see protein concentrations expressed in g l^{-1}, mg l^{-1}, μg l^{-1}, or even mg ml^{-1} (which is equivalent to g l^{-1}).

Enzymes are measured in units of activity. This is achieved by measuring how much substrate is used or product formed in a given period of time. There used to be many different enzyme units used in clinical laboratories with almost one unit for each enzyme; these had names such as King–Armstrong and Somogi units. Enzyme activities have now been standardized on the **international unit** (iu or U) and most enzymes' activities are expressed in iu. This is defined as the activity of enzyme that will catalyse 1 μmol substrate per minute under defined conditions of pH, temperature and substrate concentration. This is then expressed as an activity per unit volume of sample, for example:

$$iu\ l^{-1} \quad iu\ ml^{-1} \quad U\ l^{-1} \quad mU\ ml^{-1}$$

The SI unit of enzyme activity is the **katal** (kat). This is defined as the activity of enzyme that transforms 1 mole of substrate in 1 second. In physiological systems enzyme activities are expressed in nkat l^{-1}. International units and katals have the following relationship:

$$1\ nkat\ l^{-1} \quad = \quad 0.06\ iu\ l^{-1}$$

The standardization of **hormones** can be difficult, particularly for those hormones where a purified preparation cannot be obtained. For these hormones it is difficult to characterize the molecule and prepare a standard. In these situations the World Health Organization prepares a reference standard, against which all other standard material and assays are calibrated. Units are arbitrary international units (U) in a given volume, e.g. mU l^{-1}. These units should not be confused with international units of enzyme activity described above.

Commonly measured analytes

The most commonly measured analytes in blood samples are given in *Table 1.2*, along with the reference range for an adult and unit of measurement. Reference ranges may vary in different laboratories depending on methodology and the local population. Some analytes also vary according to the gender or age of the patient (refer to the relevant chapter of this book for more details).

Methods used in clinical biochemistry

There is a wide range of methods used in clinical biochemistry to look for many varied substances found in the blood and other biological fluids. In

Table 1.2 Commonly measures analytes in blood samples

	Analyte	Reference	Units	Chapter
Ions	Calcium	2.25–2.88	mmol l^{-1}	8
	Hydrogen	36–44	nmol l^{-1}	14
	Magnesium	0.7–1.0	mmol l^{-1}	8
	Potassium	3.6–5.0	mmol l^{-1}	7
	Sodium	135–145	mmol l^{-1}	7
	Phosphate	0.8–1.4	mmol l^{-1}	8
	Bicarbonate	22–30	mmol l^{-1}	14
Enzymes	Alkaline phosphatase	20–70	iu l^{-1}	10
	Acid phosphatase	4–11	iu l^{-1}	10
	Amylase	25–125	iu l^{-1}	10
	AST	11–26	iu l^{-1}	10
	ALT	8–30	iu l^{-1}	10
	Creatine kinase	<90	iu l^{-1}	10
Proteins	Albumin	35–50	g l^{-1}	12
	Total protein	60–80	g l^{-1}l	12
	Immunoglobulin G	6.5–13.5	g l^{-1}	15
Lipids	Cholesterol (fasting)	<5.2	mmol l^{-1}	13
	Triglyceride	0.4–1.8	mmol l^{-1}	13
Major metabolites	Creatinine	60–110	µmol l^{-1}	17
	Bilirubin	3–20	µmol l^{-1}	18
	Glucose (fasting)	2.8–6.0	mmol l^{-1}	5
	Urea	3.3–6.7	mmol l^{-1}	17
Hormones	Cortisol 09.00	140–690	nmol l^{-1}	5
	24.00	<100	nmol l^{-1}	
	Total thyroxine	60–150	nmol l^{-1}	6
	TSH	0.3–4.0	mU l^{-1}	6
Gases	Carbon dioxide	4.5–6.0	kPa	14
	Oxygen	11–15	kPa	14

this book the principles of the most important methods used in the laboratory are discussed at the end of a chapter. The particular analytical technique that is discussed has relevance to the analyte or analytes under discussion in that chapter; for instance, electrophoresis is discussed in the chapter on proteins (Chapter 12). The list below shows in which chapter particular analytical techniques are described.

Atomic absorption spectroscopy	Chapter 8
Chromatography	Chapter 11
Electrophoresis	Chapter 12
Enzyme measurements	Chapter 10
Flame emission spectroscopy	Chapter 7
Gas electrodes	Chapter 14
Immunoassays	Chapters 5 and 6
Immunoblotting	Chapter 15
Immunofixation	Chapter 15
Ion-selective electrodes	Chapter 7
Polymerase chain reaction	Chapter 4
Spectroscopy	Chapter 2

SUGGESTED FURTHER READING

Anderson S.C. and Cockayne S. (2002) *Clinical Chemistry: Concepts and Applications.* New York: McGraw-Hill Medical.

Beckett G.J., Ashby P., Rae P. and Walker S.W. (2005) *Lecture Notes on Clinical Biochemistry,* 7th edition. Oxford: Blackwell Publishing.

Burtis C.A. and Ashwood E.R. (2001) *Tietz's Fundamentals of Clinical Chemistry,* 5th edition. London: WB Saunders Co. Ltd.

Burtis C.A., Ashwood E.R. and Bruns D.E. (2005) *Tietz's Textbook of Clinical Chemistry and Molecular Diagnostics,* 4th edition. London: WB Saunders Co. Ltd.

Cook M. (2006) *Clinical Chemistry and Metabolic Medicine,* 7th edition. London: Hodder Arnold.

Gaw A., Cowan R.A., O'Reilly D.StJ., Stewart M.J. and Shepherd J. (2004) *An Illustrated Colour Text: Clinical Biochemistry,* 3rd edition. London: Elsevier Health Sciences.

Marshall W.J. and Bangert S.K. (2004) *Clinical Chemistry,* 5th edition. London: Mosby.

SELF-ASSESSMENT QUESTIONS

1. What are the main functions of a clinical biochemistry laboratory?
2. What are the analytical factors affecting the results of a biochemical test?
3. How are physiological factors that affect a biochemical test grouped?
4. Define the term reference range.
5. Define clinical sensitivity.
6. Define clinical specificity.
7. What is used to prevent blood samples clotting?
8. How would you normally express a concentration in the range of 10^{-3} M?
9. Express 0.65 nmol μl^{-1} in $\mu mol\ l^{-1}$.
10. What factors influence an enzyme reaction?

Nutrition and drugs

Learning objectives
After studying this chapter you should confidently be able to:

■ **Describe the terms macro- and micronutrients.**
Macronutrients maintain the structure, function and energy supply of the body. Micronutrients maintain the function of the cell.

■ **Review the roles of water, carbohydrate, fat and protein in the diet.**
The body must balance intake and need with output and loss. Water is required to maintain the fluid volume of the body. An average adult will drink between 1500 and 2500 ml per day. Carbohydrate balance is controlled by a complex interaction of hormones. The major function of carbohydrate is to supply energy. Fat intake is important in maintaining cell integrity, steroid hormone synthesis and energy storage. Proteins are used in many different processes in the body and are vital for the maintenance of health.

■ **Explain the need for vitamins and minerals in maintaining health.**
Vitamins, minerals and trace elements are required in small amounts and are essential for the normal regulation of metabolic activity. Diseases of nutrition relate to an excess or to a deficiency.

■ **Describe the role of the clinical biochemistry laboratory in measuring drugs.**
Drug measurements within a clinical biochemistry laboratory are to assess therapeutic levels or to determine drug overdose or abuse. Therapeutic drug monitoring enables drugs to be maintained within the therapeutic range.

■ **Calculate the concentration of a substance using simple spectrophotometric data.**
Colorimetry is the most commonly used technique to analyse patients' samples within a clinical biochemistry laboratory. The wavelength of light is measured in nanometres and a coloured substance has an absorbance maximum.

2.1 COMPOSITION OF THE BODY

To maintain health we require a minimum amount of food to supply the energy we need to live and the building blocks needed to grow and replace old cells. The amount of food we need varies from person to person depending on their body size and energy expenditure: a large manual labourer requires more energy than a small sedentary office worker. The amount of energy required each day in the diet is equivalent to the sum of energy usage by basal metabolism, physical activity and heat production. A sick person has higher energy demands than a healthy one and therefore requires increased energy input – sometimes by 100% or more for patients with burns.

Every day we need to take in water, protein, fats, carbohydrates, and a number of minerals, vitamins and trace elements. **Macronutrients** are the major components required to maintain the structure, function and energy supply of the body; these are carbohydrates, lipids and proteins. **Micronutrients** are those materials needed in small amounts to maintain cell function and these include vitamins, minerals and trace metals. Micronutrients are important to health, as many are used as cofactors or parts of enzymes required for metabolic reactions.

The general principle followed is that the body must balance intake and need with output and loss. For example, the body needs to maintain its energy balance and its water balance. If this balance is lost then a deficiency state or disease associated with excess may develop. A number of physiological factors affect nutritional requirements, including growth, gender and age (see *Box 2.1*).

Box 2.1 Basal metabolic rate

The basal metabolic rate (BMR) is the energy required by an individual at rest to maintain normal metabolic processes. This is measured while the individual is awake. Many factors influence the BMR such as age, environmental temperature, fitness and nutritional state. As a rule of thumb the BMR can be estimated for an individual adult according to the following formula:

$$BMR = Weight\ (kg) \times 100\ kJ\ day^{-1}$$

2.2 MACRONUTRIENTS

Water

Water is the most abundant material in living cells, which normally contain 65–90% water. We require water as a **solvent** in which many nutrients and waste products are dissolved and transported around the body. More importantly, water is needed to maintain the fluid volume of the body and cells, as water has a major influence on cell structure and cell function. Without water we would die in a few days, as the body would become dehydrated which leads to circulatory collapse due to the loss of fluid volume.

Water is taken in through drink and food, and is made in the body by the oxidation of various foods. The amount of water required depends on the size of the body; for an average adult this will be between 1500 and 2500 ml per day. More will be required in a hot climate or during prolonged heavy exercise. Water is lost in the urine, faeces, sweat and through the lungs as water vapour. The sum of water loss from skin and lungs is called the **insensible loss**. Visible sweat is called **sensible loss**. *Table 2.1* shows typical amounts involved in water balance.

Table 2.1 Typical amounts of water involved in the intake and loss of water for an adult

Water input		Water loss	
From drinks	1500 ml	In urine	1400 ml
From food	800 ml	In faeces	100 ml
Made in the body	200 ml	Insensible	700 ml
		Sensible	300 ml
Total	2500 ml	Total	2500 ml

Water is distributed between two compartments in the body; the **extracellular** compartment and the **intracellular** compartment. The fluid associated with each compartment is called the extracellular fluid (ECF) and the intracellular fluid (ICF), respectively. See Chapter 7 for a detailed look at water balance.

Carbohydrate

Rice, potatoes and cereal grain are the major sources of dietary carbohydrates that provide the most efficient source of energy in the form of sugars and starches. In a Western diet approximately 45% of the body's energy requirement is supplied as carbohydrate. Most of the carbohydrate is broken down and absorbed in the gut as **monosaccharides** such as glucose, fructose, galactose and mannose.

The body needs to maintain the blood glucose level to supply fuel for its metabolic processes. The brain is particularly dependent on the supply of glucose to maintain cerebral function. To do this a minimum of 150 g per day of glucose is required. Complicated mechanisms regulate blood glucose concentrations. These are described in Chapter 9.

Fats

Fats are an important part of the diet because of their high energy content, which is more than twice that of carbohydrate or protein (see *Table 2.2*). Approximately 75 g of fat is required daily. The body stores energy as fat in adipose tissue, ready to be used when the energy input does not meet the body's demands.

Fat is a term for a collection of chemicals called **lipids**, the main ones being **fatty acids**, **triglycerides** and **steroids**. Fatty acids are used in the

Table 2.2 Energy values of food

	Energy value (kJ g^{-1})	Content in diet (%)
Carbohydrate	17	46
Fat	37	42
Protein	17	12

synthesis of intermediate compounds used in many metabolic pathways and in the production of prostaglandins and other molecules important in the regulation of cell function. The diet supplies essential fatty acids which cannot be synthesized in the body, namely linoleic acid and arachidonic acid. Triglycerides are synthesized from glycerol and fatty acids and are used as high energy stores for use in times of need. Steroids share a common structure called perhydrocyclopentanophenanthrene, which is composed of four rings, three 6-carbon rings and one 5-carbon ring. Cholesterol and steroid hormones are all derivatives of this ringed skeleton. *Figure 2.1* shows the structure of the important lipids.

One of the most clinically important lipids taken in the diet is cholesterol. Practically all cells in the body contain cholesterol, which maintains the integrity of the cell wall, and without cholesterol they would not

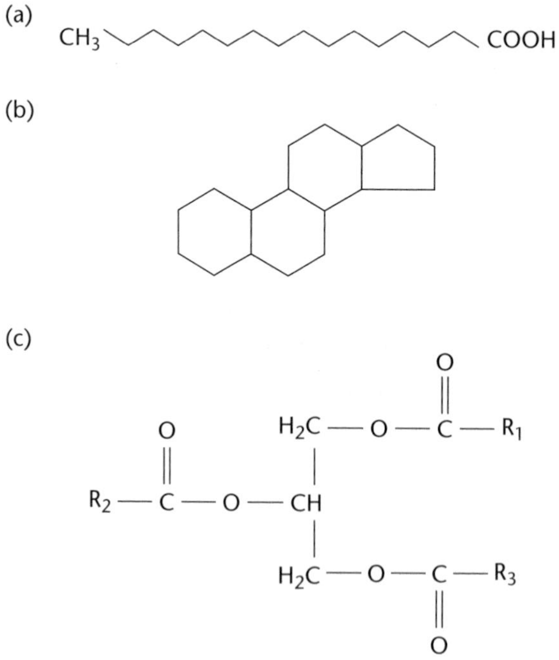

(a)

CH$_3$ ∿∿∿∿∿∿ COOH

(b)

(c)

Figure 2.1
Basic structures of the important lipids taken in the diet. (a) fatty acid; (b) steroid; (c) triglyceride.

function. However, high levels of cholesterol in the diet have been associated with a greater risk of heart disease through the development of **atheroma** (see Chapter 13).

Protein

Proteins are composed of **amino acids** which provide the building blocks to synthesize new proteins, which are constantly being removed and replaced. To maintain this process between 40 and 60 g of protein are required per day, depending on body size. Considerably more protein is required during growth, infections and following burns or trauma, when the synthesis of new protein is greater. To estimate the adequacy of protein intake, the nitrogen balance of the patient is calculated. This reflects the difference between protein intake and breakdown. Intake is given by the amount of protein in the diet and breakdown is related to the concentration of urea nitrogen (the major catabolite of protein) in the urine. A positive balance indicates a net protein synthesis whilst a negative balance indicates protein breakdown. An approximate idea of nitrogen balance can be obtained using the following formula:

$$\text{Nitrogen balance} = \frac{\text{protein intake g day}^{-1}}{6.25} - \text{urinary urea N g day}^{-1} + 3$$

Not only is there a requirement for sufficient protein but the type of protein is also important as proteins supply essential amino acids, so called because they cannot be synthesized in the body. These are shown in *Table 2.3*.

Proteins that supply all the essential amino acids are termed **complete proteins**; proteins lacking in a particular essential amino acid are **incomplete**. Animal proteins with the exception of gelatine are complete, cereal proteins lack lysine, and leguminous proteins lack methionine. A vegetarian diet should be varied to supply all the essential amino acids.

Table 2.3 The essential amino acids and typical requirements for an adult

Amino acid	Daily requirement (mg day^{-1} kg^{-1} body wt)
Histidine	Unknown
Isoleucine	12
Leucine	16
Lysine	12
Methionine	10
Phenylalanine	16
Threonine	8
Tryptophan	3
Valine	14

Box 2.2 Nutritional assessment

The nutritional assessment of a patient involves collecting dietary information, noting physical signs and measuring the height and weight. Skinfold measurements can give an estimate of the amount of body fat. Other factors such as medication, medical history and immunological status are also considered when making a full nutritional assessment.

Protein also provides an important source of nitrogen, sulphur and phosphorus for the body (see *Box 2.2*).

2.3 MICRONUTRIENTS

Vitamins

Vitamins are organic compounds required in only trace amounts for health and growth. They are naturally occurring compounds, found in animals and plants. Nowadays many can be artificially synthesized. They are important in maintaining the proper functioning of enzymes which are involved in many different processes such as the maintenance of vision, calcium metabolism, blood clotting, connective tissue formation and the normal metabolism of lipids, carbohydrates and proteins. Vitamins can be divided into two groups, **fat-soluble vitamins** and **water-soluble vitamins**. The fat-soluble vitamins, (vitamins A, D, E and K) are absorbed and stored in body tissues, mainly the liver, whereas water-soluble vitamins are lost in the urine and need continual replacement. As the fat-soluble vitamins are stored in lipid-rich organs, an abnormally high intake of these vitamins can have toxic effects (see *Box 2.3*).

Box 2.3 Vitamins

Sir Frederick Gowland (1861–1947) was the first to undertake a scientific study of vitamins. He was nearly 50 years old when he began his work on 'accessory food factors' (vitamins). He showed that rats reared on pure protein, carbohydrate, fat and water failed to grow. If a few drops of milk were also added to the diet then the rats grew. He was awarded a Nobel Prize in 1929 with another scientist, Christiaan Eijkman, who studied beriberi.

Vitamin deficiency leads to a disease state when particular metabolic processes are unable to function fully, resulting in symptoms of deficiency. The following section covers the major vitamins required for health, their role and such deficiency and toxic states that may arise; firstly the fat-soluble and then water-soluble vitamins. The recommended daily allowance (RDA) is also given.

Vitamin A

The RDA for vitamin A (retinol) is 1 mg for males and 0.8 mg for females. Vitamin A is found in fish oils and liver, and is required for vision, growth and reproduction. Deficiency results in poor night adaptation to low levels of light or night blindness (nyctalopia) and the skin becomes rough and dry with hyperkeratosis. Toxic effects can result in bone and joint pains, hair loss, anorexia, weight loss, headaches and hepatomegaly.

Vitamin D

For vitamin D (calciferols) the RDA is 10 μg while growing, then changing to 5 μg. It is found in plants and made by the action of sunlight on 7-dehydrocholesterol in the skin. Vitamin D is required for the maintenance of calcium metabolism. Deficiency results in hypocalcaemia, leading to osteomalacia in adults and rickets in children. Toxic levels lead to hypercalcaemia.

Vitamin E

The RDA for vitamin E (tocopherols) is 10 mg. Vitamin E is found in plants and vegetable oils and is required for its antioxidant properties, preventing damage from free radicals. Deficiency results in haemolytic anaemia, irritability and oedema. Toxic levels may lead to prolonged bleeding times due to vitamin E preventing the absorption of vitamin K.

Vitamin K

For vitamin K the RDA is 70–140 μg. Vitamin K is found in plants and is required for the synthesis of the clotting factors prothrombin, factor VII, factor IX and factor X. Deficiency results in defective blood coagulation, leading to haemorrhagic disease in infants. Toxic levels may lead to haemolytic anaemia.

Vitamin B$_1$

The RDA for vitamin B$_1$ (thiamin) is 1.0–1.5 mg. Vitamin B$_1$ is found in unrefined cereal grains, liver, heart and kidney. It is required as the coenzyme for transketolases. Deficiency results in beriberi, which can have symptoms of mental confusion, anorexia, muscular weakness, ataxia, oedema, muscle wasting and cardiac problems.

Vitamin B$_2$

For vitamin B$_2$ (riboflavin) the RDA is 1.2–1.7 mg. Vitamin B$_2$ is found in liver, kidney, milk and green vegetables. It is required as a coenzyme and for use in oxidation–reduction and energy-forming reactions. Deficiency results in sore throat, swollen pharyngeal and oral mucous membranes, glossitis, seborrhoeic dermatitis and anaemia.

Vitamin B$_6$

The RDA for vitamin B$_6$ (pyridoxine) is 2.0–2.2 mg. Vitamin B$_6$ is found in meats, fish, yeast and bran and also in lesser amounts in milk and eggs. It is required as a coenzyme in many enzyme reactions. Deficiency is rare but can result in convulsion, dermatitis and anaemia.

Vitamin B$_{12}$

For vitamin B$_{12}$ (cyanocobalamin) the RDA is 0.5 μg. Vitamin B$_{12}$ is found in meats, milk and eggs. It is required for the formation of active folate coenzyme. Deficiency results in megaloblastic anaemia and neuropathy, with symptoms such as weakness, paralysis, confusion and dementia. A deficiency may result from a lack of intrinsic factor, which is synthesized in the stomach and is required for the absorption of vitamin B$_{12}$ by the intestine. This gives rise to pernicious anaemia.

Vitamin C

For vitamin C (ascorbic acid) the RDA is 60 mg. Vitamin C is found in citrus fruits, blackcurrants, melons, tomatoes, green peppers and leafy green vegetables. It is required as a cofactor for protocollagen hydroxylase and for tyrosine metabolism. Deficiency results in scurvy, which is a condition where connective tissue cannot form correctly. Symptoms include swollen and tender joints, bleeding gums, cutaneous bleeding, bruising, psychological problems and sometimes anaemia (see *Box 2.4*).

Box 2.4 Scurvy

Scurvy is the disease that occurs when insufficient vitamin C is found in the diet. The symptoms seen are as a result of weakened blood vessels and damage to the capillary beds, giving slow wound healing. These are most easily seen in changes in teeth and bleeding gums. Scurvy used to be a problem for sailors on long voyages where there was no fresh fruit available. British sailors used to take lime juice to prevent scurvy, leading to the name 'limey' for British people.

Niacin

The RDA for niacin (nicotinic acid) is 18 mg. Niacin is found in meat, liver, yeast and poultry, and in lesser amounts in milk and leafy green vegetables. It is required in many enzyme reactions, for example dehydrogenase reactions. Deficiency results in pellagra, a chronic wasting disease associated with dermatitis, dementia and diarrhoea.

Folic acid

For folic acid (pteroylglutamic acid) the RDA is 200 µg. Folic acid is found in leafy green vegetables. It is required as a coenzyme for use in the metabolism of amino acids. Deficiency results in megaloblastic anaemia and sensory and neurological changes.

Biotin

The RDA for biotin is 100–200 µg for young infants. Biotin is found in liver, eggs, yeast and milk. Gut flora synthesizes biotin in adults. It is required for enzyme reactions involving carboxylases. Deficiency is rare but can result in nausea, vomiting, depression, anorexia and a dry, scaly dermatitis.

Pantothenic acid

For pantothenic acid the RDA is 4–7 mg. Pantothenic acid is found in egg yolk, kidney, liver and yeast. It is required for carbohydrate and lipid metabolism. Deficiency states are unlikely to occur in humans.

2.4 MINERALS AND TRACE ELEMENTS

Besides vitamins, the other important micronutrients necessary for health are minerals and trace elements. The more important minerals, such as calcium, will be discussed in later chapters. Only an overview of minerals and trace elements will be given here. Minerals and trace elements can be considered to be the essential, non-organic elements required for health. If the element is present in biological tissues in larger quantities (mg g^{-1} of tissue), for example phosphate or calcium, this is a **mineral**. If the element is present in smaller amounts (µg g^{-1} or less), this is considered to be a **trace element**, for example zinc. Some elements may be regarded as **ultra-trace elements** if they are found in ng g^{-1} amounts, for example gold. In terms of daily requirements, minerals are measured in g per day, trace elements in mg or µg per day.

Essential elements are those which are required for the maintenance of health and growth. There is an optimal concentration, above and below which a toxic or deficiency state may result, producing clinical symptoms. *Table 2.4* shows the essential elements, classified as a mineral or a trace element.

Trace elements are required in very small amounts to maintain health and they often form essential parts of enzymes and hormones which regulate metabolism. Thus, deficiency of a trace element will result in changes in the metabolic equilibrium as enzyme substrate accumulates, eventually leading to clinical symptoms. For example, copper is important in many metalloenzymes such as cytochrome oxidase and superoxide dismutase; a deficiency leads to connective tissue defects, lack of pigmentation and ataxia. An excess

Table 2.4 The essential elements (in order of atomic number)

Minerals	Trace elements
Sodium	Fluorine
Magnesium	Silicon
Phosphorus	Vanadium
Sulphur	Chromium
Chlorine	Manganese
Potassium	Iron
Calcium	Cobalt
	Nickel
	Copper
	Zinc
	Arsenic
	Selenium
	Molybdenum
	Iodine

of trace element is often toxic because it 'poisons' other enzyme systems or transport mechanisms (see *Box 2.5*).

Box 2.5 Ataxia

Ataxia is an inability to co-ordinate voluntary movements and the patient staggers and can appear to be under the influence of alcohol.

2.5 ASSESSMENT OF NUTRITIONAL STATUS

In most hospitals, evaluation of the nutritional status of the patient depends on dietary history, clinical assessment and measurements such as weight and skin-fold thickness. Despite this, the clinical biochemistry laboratory still plays a part in nutritional assessment. A number of biochemical tests are used in conjunction with haematological results. There are two main nutritional problems that are seen in patients referred for investigation. The first is **obesity**, a common problem today. The second is more important from the laboratory's point of view, and that is malnutrition. Malnutrition can be an overall deficit of nutritional elements such as carbohydrate and protein, or may involve a selective deficit of a particular vitamin or trace element. Blood analysis for vitamins and trace elements can help the clinician in evaluating particular patients. In the case of more generalized malnutrition, the protein intake is important as the amino acids are used to synthesize new proteins in the body. Protein deficiency arising from generalized malnutrition is called **marasmus**. Where the principal cause of malnutrition is a protein deficiency, in the presence of adequate energy intake, this is called **kwashiorkor**. The laboratory evaluation of protein deficiency can be performed by measuring the concentration of serum proteins, in particular albumin (see Chapter 12).

Malnutrition may not always be associated with lack of nutrients but may reflect other pathology occurring in the patient, for example, malabsorption and protein-losing conditions. Diseases that are associated with malabsorption are discussed in the next chapter.

2.6 TOXICOLOGY

Besides taking in nutrients we can also take in drugs and toxic substances. The clinical biochemistry laboratory is often required to make an assessment of drug levels in patients to help monitor therapy or to investigate a suspected case of drug overdose or poisoning. We can consider these two situations separately when considering drug analysis in the laboratory.

Therapeutic drug monitoring

Therapeutic drug monitoring is the measurement of drug levels in a patient's blood sample taken after a defined time, allowing adjustment of therapy to be made if necessary. Many factors are involved in the metabolism of drugs, including the rate of absorption, distribution of the drug within the body compartments, distribution between free drug and protein-bound drug, biotransformation of the drug by metabolizing enzymes and the rate of excretion. Consequently, for a given dose of drug taken, different individuals will have quite different concentrations of drug in their blood after a given time period.

Table 2.5 Some therapeutic drugs commonly monitored in the clinical biochemistry laboratory

Anticonvulsants
Phenobarbitone
Phenytoin
Sodium valporate
Carbamazepine
Digoxin
Theophylline
Lithium
Methotrexate
Cyclosporine

Many therapeutic drugs need to reach a minimum concentration in the blood before they are effective, and this concentration is called **the minimum effective concentration** (MEC). If too much drug is given, the patient may suffer from toxic side effects. The concentration of drug above which toxic effects are noted is called the **minimum toxic concentration** (MTC). The concentration range between the MEC and MTC is called the **therapeutic range** or **therapeutic window**. Fluctuating levels of drug are found in blood samples, depending on the time elapsed between drug ingestion and when the sample was taken. This is seen in *Fig. 2.2*. For some drugs, the therapeutic range is small and the level of drug in the blood must be tightly controlled to be effective but not have toxic side effects.

Drug overdose

Occasionally the clinical biochemistry department will be called upon to perform urgent analysis on blood specimens from patients with a suspected drug overdose. Drugs such as salicylate (aspirin), paracetamol, barbiturates or iron tablets may have been taken either deliberately or accidentally. An urgent measurement of the suspected drug will confirm an overdose and aid the treatment given to the patient. Urgent measurements are only offered for certain drugs where knowledge of the drug level would influence the treatment, for example, where there is an antidote or a particular treatment regime is prescribed.

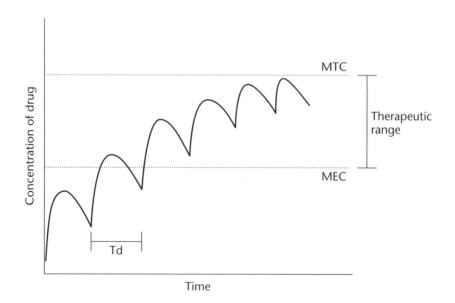

Figure 2.2
Fluctuating drug concentration in a blood sample. Td is the time between doses, MEC is the minimum effective concentration and MTC is the minimum toxic concentration.

Some laboratories will screen urine sample for drugs of abuse, which include morphine and morphine analogues, amphetamine, methadone and phenobarbital.

2.7 LABORATORY MEASUREMENT OF NUTRIENTS AND DRUGS

Nutritional assessment of macronutrients is usually by physical examination and from the nutritional history of the patient. Minerals are often measured within the clinical biochemistry laboratory but not usually as an investigation of nutritional status, rather as an investigation into other diseases (these methods are covered in other chapters). Micronutrients, on the other hand, are sometimes measured in specialized centres to assess nutritional status. Within the clinical biochemistry laboratory the elements of nutritional and toxicological intake are performed by a wide range of techniques, from simple colour reactions to analytical methods using expensive and sophisticated instrumentation. Vitamins can be measured **spectrophotometrically**, by enzyme reactions requiring the vitamin as a cofactor, by **immunoassays** and by **chromatography**. Trace metals are analysed and measured using **atomic absorption spectroscopy**, as discussed in greater detail in Chapter 8. Many drugs are measured and identified by rapid immunochemical techniques as discussed in Chapters 5 and 6, and by chromatography, as discussed in Chapter 11.

Some of the earliest methods for measuring vitamins and drugs involved the formation of coloured products in a chemical reaction, and some of these methods are still used today, especially for quick screening tests. The intensity of the colour is measured by colorimetry and related to the concentration of the test vitamin or drug. Some examples of colorimetric measurements are given in *Table 2.6*.

Table 2.6 Some compounds which can be measured by colorimetry, the colour of the product and the wavelength at which the absorbance is measured

Compound	Reactant	Colour produced	Wavelength measured (nm)
Vitamin A	Trifluoroacetic acid	Blue	620
Vitamin C	2,4-Dinitrophenyl hydrazine	Red/purple	520
Salicylates	Ferric ions	Violet	540
Bilirubin	Diazotized sulphanilic acid	Blue	600
Protein	Cuprous ions	Reddish–violet	540
Creatinine	Picrate	Red–orange	500

2.8 SPECTROSCOPY AND COLORIMETRY

The most common technique used within a laboratory to measure the concentration of an analyte is spectrophotometry, which is the measurement of the intensity of a colour formed by a chemical or enzymatic reaction. It would be true to say that most measurements made in the clinical biochemistry laboratory involve the formation of a colour, the intensity of which is proportional to the concentration of the analyte in question. Commonly, the measurement of colour intensity is called **colorimetry** and is performed at a single wavelength. A narrow band-pass filter is used to select the required wavelength (see *Box 2.6*).

Box 2.6 Light

Light is electromagnetic radiation of a particular frequency and wavelength. The visible spectrum lies between about 400 nm and 700 nm, giving violet and red light, respectively. The wavelengths of other colours are given below:

Violet	400 nm
Blue	460 nm
Green	500 nm
Yellow	570 nm
Orange	600 nm
Red	700 nm

A coloured solution will absorb light of a particular wavelength, allowing the other wavelengths to pass through the solution and be detected, by eye or electronically. This means that a red solution **absorbs blue light** allowing the red light to pass through – which we see and recognize as red. Conversely, a blue solution will absorb red light.

Spectroscopy is different to colorimetry in that the wavelength of light passing through a sample of coloured solution is continually changed. *Figure 2.3a* shows a simplified diagram of a spectrophotometer that uses a prism to select or change the wavelength of light passing through the sample. The amount of light absorbed for each wavelength is measured to produce an **absorption spectrum** for that solution; *Fig. 2.3b* shows an example of this. This is performed on a **spectrophotometer**, which uses a prism or a grating to split white light into its component wavelengths. For colorimetric methods used in the laboratory, the absorption spectrum of the coloured product has previously been determined and the wavelength where the maximum absorption occurs is used in the test. Colorimeters are simple instruments that use filters to select the desired wavelength.

The amount of light absorbed is given in **absorbance** units (also called the **optical density**): the higher the reading, the greater the absorbance and the more intense the colour of the solution. The absorbance is related to the concentration of coloured compound in solution according to the formula, referred to as Beer's law:

$$A = \varepsilon\, l\, c$$

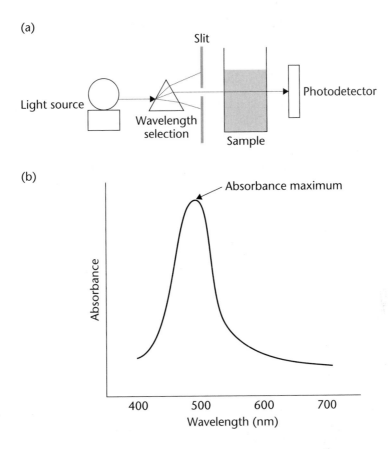

Figure 2.3
(a) Diagrammatic representation of a simple spectrophotometer where wavelength selection is achieved by rotating the prism. An absorbance spectrum is obtained (b) by measuring the absorbance at each wavelength

where A = absorbance; ε = molar extinction coefficient (sometimes referred to as molar absorption coefficient); l = pathlength; and c = concentration of coloured compound (in mol l^{-1})

The molar extinction coefficient is a constant for the coloured compound at a given wavelength; it is the absorbance given by 1 mole of the compound and indicates how efficiently the compound absorbs light energy. The pathlength is the distance the light travels through the sample and is constant for any measurement, usually 1 cm. This leaves the concentration term variable, and thus:

$$A \propto c$$

Some methods relate absorbance directly to the concentration but it is more usual to run a standard or series of standards of known concentrations to calibrate the method. If the absorbance of a standard (known concentration) and a test is measured then the concentration of the unknown can be found using the formula:

$$\text{Concentration of unknown} = \frac{\text{absorbance of test}}{\text{absorbance of standard}} \times \text{concentration of standard}$$

It is necessary to take an absorbance reading of a sample with no analyte present (**blank reading**) and subtract this value from all other readings; this is often automatic in many laboratory analysers. Although the majority of absorbance measurements are made in the visible region of the spectrum, there are some applications where absorbance is measured in the ultra-violet region. The measurement of a number of drugs, for example barbiturates, can be made from the UV absorption spectrum of the drug. Most UV measurements are associated with enzymes (see Chapter 10). There are some specialized applications where an infrared spectrum is used to determine the composition of renal stones (see *Box 2.7*).

Box 2.7 Salicylate overdose

A 25-year-old male was brought into A&E suspected of taking a drug overdose. Blood was taken and analysed for salicylate. The plasma gave an optical density of 0.9 and a 100 mg l^{-1} standard gave an optical density of 0.55. The optical densities had a blank value subtracted. The patient had a plasma salicylate of:

$$\frac{0.9}{0.55} \times 100 = 164 \text{ mg l}^{-1}$$

This is a high salicylate level but not life-threatening: levels greater than 300 mg l^{-1} give toxic symptoms and levels greater than 600 mg l^{-1} can be fatal. An overdose of salicylate can give rise to a complex acid–base disturbance resulting in hyperventilation (see Chapter 14), tinnitus and headaches.

SUGGESTED FURTHER READING

In addition to relevant chapters in the textbooks cited in Chapter 1 the following references are recommended.

Bates C.J. (1997) Vitamin analysis. *Annals of Clinical Biochemistry*, **34**: 599–626.
Bogdon J.D., ed. (2000) *Clinical Nutrition of the Essential Trace Elements and Minerals: The Guide for Health Professionals (Nutrition & Health)*. Totowa, NJ: Humana Press Inc.
Burton M., Schentag J.J., Evans W. and Shaw L. (2005) *Applied Pharmacokinetics and Pharmacodynamics: Principles of Therapeutic Drug Monitoring*, 4th edition. Philadelphia: Lippincott Williams & Wilkins.
Philippsborn H. (2005) *Elsevier's Dictionary of Vitamins and Pharmacochemistry*. London: Elsevier.
Rosenfeld L. (1997). Vitamine–vitamin. The early years of discovery. *Clinical Chemistry*, **43**: 680–685.

Taylor A. (1996) Detection and monitoring of disorders of essential trace elements. *Annals of Clinical Biochemistry*, **33**: 486–510.

Thomas D.R. (2004) Vitamins in health and aging. *Clinics in Geriatric Medicine*, **20**: 259–274.

SELF-ASSESSMENT QUESTIONS

1. What are the three major macronutrients?
2. What are the three classes of micronutrients?
3. Which diseases are associated with insufficient protein in the diet?
4. Which are the four water-soluble vitamins?
5. In general, what concentration should a drug have to be clinically effective?
6. Which technique measures the colour produced in a chemical reaction?
7. How is spectroscopy different from colorimetry?
8. Given that bilirubin has a molar extinction coefficient of 60 700 at 453 nm, what is the molar concentration of a solution of bilirubin that has an absorbance of 0.50?
9. Given that a 100 mg l^{-1} standard of salicylate gave an absorbance of 0.75 in a salicylate test, what is the concentration of salicylate in a sample that gives an absorbance of 0.35?

Digestion

Learning objectives
After studying this chapter you should confidently be able to:

■ **Describe the digestive process for macronutrients.**
   The stomach secretes acid, pepsin and intrinsic factor. Acidic chyme is
   neutralized in the duodenum. Pancreatic juice and succus entericus are
   the major sources of digestive enzymes. Water-soluble nutrients are
   absorbed through microvilli on the intestinal epithelial cells and fats and
   glycerol are absorbed through the lacteals of the villus. Bile is necessary
   for the absorption of fats.

■ **List and describe the function of the important gut hormones.**
   Gut hormones control the digestive process by regulating enzyme
   secretion, gut movement and the release of other gut hormones. The
   important hormones include gastrin, secretin, CCK-PZ, VIP and GIP.
   Gastrin produced in the stomach is regulated by the hydrogen ion
   concentration of the stomach. Uncontrolled gastrin secretion can lead to
   Zollinger–Ellison syndrome.

■ **Give examples of tests used to investigate malabsorption.**
   Malabsorption can be assessed through the measurement of faecal fat.
   Elevated serum amylase levels are found in pancreatitis.

In order to be of benefit, food containing all the elements of nutrition must
be taken into the body, broken down and absorbed; this is called **digestion.**
Assuming a sufficient intake of food to meet the needs of the body, we will
maintain our regular metabolic processes. These can be upset and result in
ill health if we do not take in sufficient food (malnutrition), or if there is a
problem in the absorption of food (malabsorption). The food we eat is a
complex mixture of protein, carbohydrate and fat that can only be absorbed
by the body when it has been broken down into its basic units, and this is
achieved by enzymes found in the digestive tract.

3.1 THE FOOD WE EAT

Proteins

Proteins are composed of long chains of amino acids joined by peptide bonds that can be broken by enzymes called proteases. Pepsin is produced in the stomach by the action of hydrochloric acid on pepsinogen and it breaks proteins into shorter peptides by splitting the peptide bonds of amino acids with aromatic side chains. Trypsin, elastase, carboxypeptidase and chymotrypsin, produced from proenzymes found in pancreatic fluid, break these peptides further. Amino acids are absorbed directly in the small intestine and short peptides can be further broken down by endopeptidase and aminopeptidase, found at the luminal surface of intestinal epithelial cells. Some peptides are absorbed via special transport mechanisms and are then hydrolysed into amino acids within the intestinal cells.

Carbohydrate

Carbohydrate taken in the diet is in the form of either **complex** or **simple carbohydrate**. Simple carbohydrates are simple sugars such as glucose, sucrose or maltose. Complex carbohydrates, such as starch and glycogen, are long chains of sugars joined together by glycosidic bonds, and may contain many branches. Complex carbohydrates are broken down by enzymes to release smaller sugars, which can be absorbed in the gut. Starch is hydrolysed to maltose by amylase, secreted by the salivary glands into the mouth.

Fat

The 60–150 g of fat taken in the diet of an average man is more than 90% triglyceride, with the remainder being cholesterol, phospholipids and free fatty acids. In the gut, fat is emulsified by bile salts that allow lipase to break the fat down to fatty acids and monoglycerides. **Micelles** are formed, allowing the transport of digested lipid to the surface of the epithelial cells lining the gut, where the lipid is absorbed.

3.2 THE DIGESTIVE PROCESS

The digestive process takes place in the alimentary canal and starts in the mouth where food is mechanically crushed by chewing and mixed with saliva containing amylase. Chewed food is swallowed and enters the stomach, which contains hydrochloric acid and pepsin. The strong muscular wall of the stomach helps to mix the food and ensure that acid and pepsin are evenly distributed. The stomach also produces a substance called intrinsic factor, necessary for the absorption of vitamin B_{12}. After about 2 hours the stomach contents (now called **chyme**) are released into the first part of the small intestine, called the duodenum (see *Box 3.1*).

Box 3.1 Gastric digestion

In 1822, at Fort Mackinac in Michigan, a Canadian trapper was involved in an accident with a duck-gun, sustaining bad abdominal wounds and a perforated stomach. William Beaumont, an American surgeon, saved the trapper's life but he was left with a fistula. Over the next 10 years, Beaumont studied digestion and gastric juice, which could easily be obtained through the trapper's fistula, making over 200 observations and giving a firm foundation to the physiology of gastric digestion.

In the duodenum the acid chyme is neutralized by pancreatic fluid entering the duodenum via the sphincter of Oddi. Pancreatic fluid is the source of the digestive enzymes trypsin, chymotrypsin, carboxypeptidase, amylase and lipase. Bile, produced by the liver and stored in the gall bladder, is also released into the gut along with pancreatic fluid. Cells lining the duodenum also produce a digestive fluid called **succus entericus**, which contains the enzymes enterokinase, peptidase, lipase, sucrase, maltase and lactase. Enterokinase activates trypsinogen to trypsin, which in turn activates chymotrypsinogen to chymotrypsin. The enzymes released into the gut continue the breakdown of food. *Table 3.1* summarizes the digestive enzymes.

Digested food is slowly passed through the small intestine, from the duodenum to the jejunum to the ileum and then to the large intestine by muscular contractions of the gut called peristalsis. The inside surface of the gut is covered with minute projections called villi, and the epithelial cells on the surface of the villi have a 'brush border' consisting of microvilli. The

Table 3.1 The digestive enzymes that act on the macronutrients and the sites of their action

Category of food	Enzyme	Site of action
Protein	Pepsin	Stomach
	Trypsin	Small intestine
	Chymotrypsin	Small intestine
	Carboxypeptidases	Small intestine
	Elastase	Small intestine
Fats	Lipase	Stomach, small intestine
	Esterase	Small intestine
	Phospholipase	Small intestine
Carbohydrates	Amylase	Mouth, small intestine
	Sucrase	Small intestine
	Maltase	Small intestine
	Lactase	Small intestine
	Trehalase	Small intestine

presence of villi and microvilli increases the surface area of the gut lining through which absorption of digested food can occur.

The majority of nutrients are absorbed in the small intestine through the surface of the villi and into the blood. Fatty acids and glycerol are absorbed into the lacteals of the villus. The blood carries nutrients to the liver where they are processed.

From the small intestine the digested food passes into the large intestine, which is divided into the caecum, the ascending colon, the transverse colon, the descending colon, and the rectum and the anal canal, where it terminates. Water and some minerals are absorbed in the large intestine, and some minerals such as iron are secreted into the large intestine. Solid waste matter is eliminated as faeces via the anus.

3.3 GUT HORMONES

The gut is also the site of production for a number of hormones that control release of digestive enzymes and the motility of the gut. The major hormones are listed below (also see *Box 3.2*).

Gastrin: produced in the stomach and stimulates the production of gastric juice, pancreatic juice and bile. Gastrin also increases intestinal motility and mucosa growth. Its production in the stomach is stimulated by a fall in stomach hydrogen ion concentration.

Secretin: produced in the duodenum and stimulates the production of pancreatic juice and insulin. Gastrin release is inhibited and there is also a reduction in gastric and duodenal mobility.

Cholecystokinin-pancreozymin (CCK-PZ): produced in the duodenum and the jejunum. This hormone regulates contractions of the gall bladder, stimulates secretion of pancreatic juice and increases small intestine motility.

Vasoactive intestinal polypeptide (VIP): produced throughout the gut and causes the relaxation of smooth muscle and the release of hormones from the pancreas, gut and hypothalamus. It increases the secretion of water and electrolytes into the gut and inhibits release of gastrin and gastric juice.

Gastric inhibitory polypeptide (GIP): produced by the duodenum and the jejunum. This hormone stimulates the release of insulin, inhibits gastric secretion and reduces intestinal mobility.

Box 3.2 The start of endocrinology

Ernest Starling (1866–1927) carried out much work on digestion and was a pioneer of endocrinology. Together with W.M. Bayliss, he discovered peristaltic waves in the intestine. Later, in 1902, they showed that a chemical messenger, released from the duodenum, stimulates the pancreas to produce pancreatic digestive juice. They subsequently called this secretin. In 1905 Starling called these biochemical messengers carried in the blood **hormones** (from the Greek word to excite – *hormeo*).

3.4 CLINICAL DISORDERS

Efficient digestion and absorption of food requires a fully functioning stomach, gall bladder and pancreas, a normal gut lining, normal peristaltic movement and normal endocrine regulation. This is a complicated association of a number of organs, each having its own role to play in the digestion and absorption of nutrients. This degree of complexity means that there is a wide range of conditions that can affect the digestive system. Most conditions only affect one organ but the effects are more far-reaching, often resulting in **maldigestion** and **malabsorption**. Diseases affecting the digestive system can be divided into three major groups:

- Infections and inflammation;
- Tumours;
- Genetic diseases.

Each of these can affect the major organs listed below:

- Stomach;
- Intestine;
- Pancreas;
- Gall bladder.

In the following section, we shall take each of the above organs in turn and discuss the various biochemical tests performed to assess the function of the organ and to investigate associated diseases.

Stomach

There are two important parameters to assess pathology associated with the stomach, and these are **stomach acid** (hydrogen ion concentration) and plasma **gastrin**. Excessive acid excretion is found in patients with peptic ulcers and gastrin-secreting tumours (**Zollinger–Ellison syndrome**) and reduced levels are found in patients with gastric cancer.

The hydrogen ion concentration of gastric juice can be measured on samples taken via a tube passed into the stomach. Where low levels of acid are found, the test can be repeated after stimulation of the stomach by **pentagastrin**. The pentagastrin stimulation test is not used very often these days but can be useful in assessing **achlorhydria** (lack of stomach acid). More commonly used is the measurement of plasma gastrin which is useful in differentiating the causes of acid hypersecretion in the stomach. Levels of plasma gastrin are measured on fasting blood samples. Reduced levels are found in patients with a peptic ulcer. High levels of gastrin and stomach acid are found in patients with Zollinger–Ellison syndrome. This is because gastrin is a hormone released in response to reduced acid levels in the stomach and a gastrin-secreting tumour does not respond to normal feedback control (see Chapter 5 for more information on feedback control of hormones). Gastrin levels are also elevated in cases of achlorhydria or hypochlorhydria as found in patients with gastritis and pernicious anaemia. A summary of the above information is given in *Table 3.2*.

Table 3.2 Changes seen in acid secretion and gastrin levels in cases of peptic ulcers, Zollinger–Ellison syndrome and gastritis

	Acid secretion	Gastrin
Ulcer	↑	↓
Zollinger–Ellison syndrome	↑	↑

Recently it was found that a major cause of a gastric ulcer is an infection with *Helicobacter pylori* which lives in the gastric mucosa. One important feature of this bacterium is that it breaks down urea to ammonia and carbon dioxide in the stomach. A number of tests have been developed to detect the presence of the bacterium by measuring ammonia or radiolabelled carbon dioxide in the breath of the patient after ingestion of urea.

Intestine

The major finding in intestinal disease is malabsorption; this may be a generalized malabsorption or of a specific dietary component such as amino acids or a certain sugar. The important diseases associated with the intestine are coeliac disease where there is a loss of surface area of the gut as a result of gluten sensitivity, gastroenteritis and tumours. A rare condition is a disaccharidase deficiency that prevents the breakdown of oligosaccharides to simple sugars, thus preventing their absorption. Investigation of intestinal disease is usually limited to the investigation of malabsorption in a routine clinical laboratory (see below). More specialized tests are performed on tissue biopsies in specialist centres.

Pancreas

The pancreas is essential for the absorption of proteins, lipids and carbohydrates as the pancreatic juice contains many digestive enzymes. Disease of the pancreas can result in malabsorption, and any disorder which interrupts the flow of pancreatic juice will impair absorption and cause a back pressure that forces pancreatic enzymes into the blood. An important investigation of the pancreas is the measurement of serum amylase. This is often an urgent investigation performed on patients admitted to A&E with stomach pain. High levels of amylase in the blood and urine are commonly associated with pancreatitis but can also be present if the patient has a pancreatic tumour. The reference range for amylase is 25–125 iu l^{-1}.

Other tests of pancreatic function involve taking samples of pancreatic fluid from the pancreatic duct via a tube passed through the stomach. Measurements of bicarbonate concentration, trypsin and amylase activity are made on the samples following stimulation by secretin or CCK-PZ. A normal response is an elevation in the measured parameters. Pancreatic disease, especially tumour of the head of pancreas, results in no stimulation or even a reduction in the levels of bicarbonate and activity of pancreatic enzymes. The volume of pancreatic juice is also an important indicator of pancreatic function following stimulation.

Gall bladder

The gall bladder, part of the hepatobiliary system, releases bile into the intestine, which is important for the absorption of fats. The bile salts present help break up the fat and form micelles. Tests for diseases associated with the hepatobiliary system are discussed in Chapter 18.

3.5   INVESTIGATION OF MALABSORPTION

The investigation of malabsorption is complicated as a number of organs are involved in the digestive process (as discussed previously). A defect in any one of the organs required for digestion and absorption (the stomach, intestine, pancreas or the hepatobiliary system) can result in malabsorption. *Table 3.3* gives examples of diseases that can result in malabsorption and the dietary component affected.

Table 3.3 Examples of various diseases which can result in malabsorption

Disease	Dietary component affected
Coeliac disease	All
Liver disease	Lipid
Pancreatitis	All
Zollinger–Ellison syndrome	Lipid
Disaccharidase deficiency	Carbohydrate

There are many tests for investigating malabsorption but often these do not directly involve the biochemistry laboratory. One test that is commonly performed in the routine clinical biochemistry laboratory is the faecal fat determination. This test measures the amount of fat excreted over a 3- or 5-day period. A timed faecal collection is homogenized and a sample of known weight (a few grams) is taken. The fat is extracted into an organic solvent, the amount present being determined by a manual titration. This is one of the few examples in a clinical biochemistry laboratory where a manual titration is performed. Normally the amount of fat excreted would not exceed 5 g per day, but this may be greatly increased in cases of malabsorption. Due to the unpleasant nature of the test, many laboratories are reluctant to perform it.

Other tests of absorption are those where a known amount of a substance is given orally and, after a sufficient time, its level is measured in the blood or urine. A good example of this type of test is the xylose absorption test. A 5 g dose of xylose is given, which is absorbed and does not undergo any metabolic processing. At least 1.5 g should appear in the urine within 5 hours. The xylose absorption test is not commonly performed as biopsies can give more information, especially regarding the presence of enzymes or transport mechanisms in the tissue.

SUGGESTED FURTHER READING

In addition to relevant chapters in the text books cited in Chapter 1 the following references are recommended.

Goldberg D.M. and Durie P.R. (1993) Biochemical tests in the diagnosis of chronic pancreatitis and in the evaluation of pancreatic insufficiency evaluation. *Biochemistry*, **26**: 253–275.
Hodgson H. and Epstein O. (2007) Malabsorption. *Medicine*, **35**: 220–225.
Lawson N. and Chestner I. (1994) Tests of exocrine pancreatic function. *Annals of Clinical Biochemistry*, **31**: 304–314.
Witt H., Apte M.V., Keim V. and Wilson J.S. (2007) Chronic pancreatitis: challenges and advances in pathogenesis, genetics, diagnosis, and therapy. *Gastroenterology*, **132**: 1557–1573.
Yadav D., Agarwal N. and Pitchumoni C.S. (2002) A critical evaluation of laboratory tests in acute pancreatitis. *American Journal of Gastroenterology*, **97**: 1309–1318.

SELF-ASSESSMENT QUESTIONS

1. Where is pepsin made?
2. Where is succus entericus synthesized?
3. Where are the majority of nutrients absorbed?
4. Where in the intestinal tract are the disaccacharidases found?
5. What stimulates the release of gastrin?
6. Which gastric hormone stimulates the release of insulin?
7. List the major organs required for normal digestion.
8. Which hormone is abnormally secreted in Zollinger–Ellison syndrome?
9. Which enzyme is a useful test for pancreatitis?
10. Which non-metabolized substance can be used in an absorption test?

Genetic control

Learning objectives
After studying this chapter you should confidently be able to:

■ **Explain how genetic information is stored and how the amino acid sequence of a protein is coded by DNA.**
DNA is double stranded and is made from the association of two strands with complementary bases forming hydrogen bonds: adenine pairs with thymine and cytosine pairs with guanine. The information required to synthesize a protein is contained in the sequence of bases of the DNA making up the particular gene. The nucleotide bases are arranged in a triplet called a codon that codes for a particular amino acid. Some codons act as a start or stop signal for protein transcription.

■ **Describe the various agents that induce DNA damage.**
Certain viruses, chemicals and a range of physical agents such as ionizing radiation, ultraviolet light and heat can cause damage to DNA. Damage to DNA can cause mutant proteins to be formed that may result in the development of cancer.

■ **Briefly describe how cancer arises as a result of the generation of oncogenes and the loss of tumour suppressor genes.**
Normal genes associated with cell division are called proto-oncogenes. Mutated genes that lead to cancer are called oncogenes. Tumour suppressor genes prevent cells from dividing, allowing time to repair damaged DNA.

■ **Explain how the polymerase chain reaction can be used to detect mutated genes.**
Molecular biology techniques for analysing DNA are becoming more common in the clinical biochemistry laboratory. The polymerase chain reaction (PCR) is a very powerful technique for identifying specific sequences of DNA from a very small sample. PCR works by amplifying a piece of DNA between two known sequences, identified by two primers. Oncogenes and oncogene products are being investigated as potential tumour markers.

In this section of the book we will study how important body functions and metabolic processes are controlled and the pathological consequences if this control is lost or altered. This chapter looks at the fundamental control of a cell – **genetic control**; and the next five chapters study different aspects of

chemical control and how different metabolic pathways are controlled by hormones secreted by endocrine tissues.

All the biochemical processes that the cell performs to maintain life and to reproduce are carefully controlled by a complex web of interactions between protein molecules within the cell. These interactions form the basis of cell signalling and synthetic pathways that direct the cell to make new products for export or cell division. In certain situations the signalling pathway directs the cell to undergo 'self-destruction' or **apoptosis**. Many metabolic pathways within the cell use enzymes to produce a product that in turn is the substrate for another enzyme. The activity of these enzymes is regulated by a number of mechanisms such as the availability of the substrate, the concentration of product or the presence of other molecules that can switch enzymes 'on' and 'off'.

Ultimately the production of all proteins, including structural proteins, cell signalling proteins and enzymes is controlled from information stored in the genes. Genes hold the genetic information essential for the smooth running of the cell. When the genetic information becomes corrupt, the normal running of the cell is disrupted and a disease process can become apparent. Increasingly, clinical biochemistry laboratories have an important role to play in the screening and diagnosis of genetic disease.

4.1 DNA AND GENETIC INFORMATION

The structure of each protein is coded for on a piece of **deoxyribonucleic acid** (DNA) called a gene. The DNA contained in a fertilized human egg only weighs about three picograms (3×10^{-12} g), i.e. 0.000000000003 g. This DNA holds all the inherited, genetic information needed to produce a new individual, controlling many factors such as height, hair colour, eye colour, size of nose and predisposition to disease in later life, for example heart disease or even cancer. The information carried by DNA is translated into the many thousands of different proteins found in the body (see *Box 4.1*).

Box 4.1 Discovery of the structure of DNA

James Watson and Francis Crick produced the first correct model of DNA in 1953, based on X-ray defraction studies by Rosalind Franklin. Their work showed how DNA could replicate, and they received the Nobel Prize in Medicine in 1962.

DNA is made from a backbone of deoxyribose molecules linked together by phosphodiester bonds. Also linked to each deoxyribose sugar is one of four nucleotide bases: **adenine, cytosine, guanine** or **thymine** (see *Fig. 4.1*). This single strand of DNA pairs with a complementary strand of DNA to form the well-known double helix. Nucleotide bases on one strand form hydrogen bonds with a **complementary** base on the other strand so that

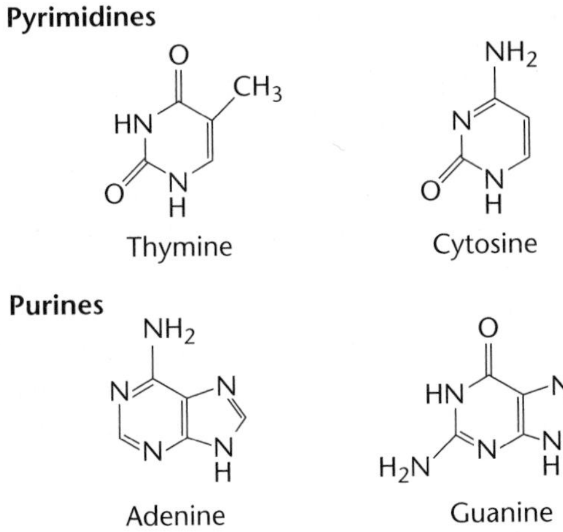

Pyrimidines

Thymine

Cytosine

Purines

Adenine

Guanine

Figure 4.1
The four bases that make up DNA.

adenine binds with thymine and **guanine binds with cytosine.** These hydrogen bonds hold the double helix together. A sequence of bases on one strand of DNA will therefore have a complementary sequence on the other strand.

Double-stranded DNA is folded around nucleoproteins, forming chromatin that condenses to form distinct chromosomes when the cell divides. During cell division a copy of the chromosome is made, the chromosomes separate and the cell splits, forming two new cells, each containing an identical copy of the genetic information. In humans there are 46 chromosomes of varying sizes: 22 pairs of somatic chromosomes and 2 sex chromosomes. During cell division, the chromosomes can be photographed and grouped together to produce a karyotype which is useful in identifying a number of genetic diseases, such as Down syndrome which is caused by an extra copy of chromosome 21 (trisomy 21).

4.2 PROTEINS FROM DNA

The genetic information to synthesize a particular protein is contained in the sequence of nucleotide bases of the DNA in the gene for the protein. There are specific nucleotide sequences that mark the start of the gene and other sequences which signal the end of the gene. In human genes there are parts of the DNA not used for protein synthesis that are not expressed; these regions interrupt the main sequence and are known as **introns**. The sequences of DNA that are expressed and used to make the protein are called **exons**.

Each protein is made from a string of amino acids, each one being coded for by a triplet of nucleotide bases on the DNA. There are two stages in synthesizing the new protein from the genetic information contained in the gene. The first is **transcription**, which involves the production of messenger ribonucleic acid (mRNA) which is a complementary copy of the sequence of bases on the DNA. mRNA is synthesized using one strand of the DNA as a template for the complementary bases that make up mRNA. The process starts at particular sites on the DNA under the control of the enzyme RNA polymerase. The RNA strand has **uracil** as the complementary base to adenine and not thymine as in DNA.

Once mRNA has been synthesized it undergoes a process called splicing. This involves the introns being removed and the exons are then spliced together (see *Fig. 4.2*). This process occurs in the nucleus under the control of enzymes in spliceosomes.

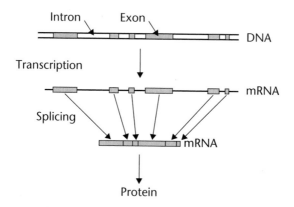

Figure 4.2
Diagram showing the bringing together of exons during transcription and splicing of mRNA.

Now the mRNA is, in effect, a copy of the information needed to synthesize the protein. Each triplet of nucleotide bases, known as a **codon**, codes for a single amino acid; this is the **genetic code** that enables 20 amino acids to be encoded by a sequence of three bases. As there are 64 combinations of three from four bases, there is redundancy in the code, and so some amino acids can be coded for by more than one codon, as shown in *Table 4.1*. Some codons act as 'punctuation', namely the three STOP codons that terminate protein synthesis. In some situations the sequence AUG, which codes for the amino acid methionine, also acts as a START signal (see *Box 4.2*).

Box 4.2 Genetic code

By 1961, Sydney Brenner and James Watson had identified the triple base pair units known as codons. The codons formed the basis for the genetic code, which was established by Har Gobind Khorana in the 1960s. Each of the 64 combinations of base pairs code for a different amino acid or a stop signal.

Table 4.1 Table of amino acids derived from codons*

First base (5′)		Middle base				Last base (3′)
		U	**C**	**A**	**G**	
First base (5′)	U	Phe	Ser	Tyr	Cys	U
		Phe	Ser	Tyr	Cys	C
		Leu	Ser	STOP	STOP	A
		Leu	Ser	STOP	Trp	G
	C	Leu	Pro	His	Arg	U
		Leu	Pro	His	Arg	C
		Leu	Pro	Gln	Arg	A
		Leu	Pro	Gln	Arg	G
	A	Ile	Thr	Asn	Ser	U
		Ile	Thr	Asn	Ser	C
		Ile	Thr	Lys	Arg	A
		Met	Thr	Lys	Arg	G
	G	Val	Ala	Asp	Gly	U
		Val	Ala	Asp	Gly	C
		Val	Ala	Glu	Gly	A
		Val	Ala	Glu	Gly	G

*For example, the codon made from the three-base sequence CGG codes for the amino acid arginine (Arg).

Following processing of the mRNA transcript, the second stage in protein synthesis occurs; this is **translation**, the process where mRNA is 'read' by ribosomes. At the ribosome a specific transfer RNA (tRNA) binds to mRNA via an **anticodon**, which is a complementary RNA triplet of bases to a codon on the mRNA. The tRNA also carries an amino acid residue (aminoacyl-tRNA) for incorporation into the new protein being synthesized. Apart from a few exceptions, there is a separate tRNA for each amino acid being used. The amino acid residue is transferred from tRNA to the growing peptide chain that eventually becomes the new protein molecule. The sequence of amino acids in the protein is the primary structure. As the protein grows it starts to fold and take on its secondary and tertiary structures, and it is this that gives the molecule its characteristic shape and enables it to perform its particular function, for example as a structural protein or an enzyme. Protein sequences are published using a single-letter code for each amino acid, as shown in *Table 4.2*.

It is important to realize that the sequence of amino acids in the protein affects the final three-dimensional shape of the molecule and is thus essential for the function of that protein. If for any reason the sequence of amino acids is disturbed or altered, then there is the possibility that the protein will

Table 4.2 Single-letter code for the amino acids

Alanine	A	Leucine	L
Arginine	R	Lysine	K
Asparagine	N	Methionine	M
Aspartic acid	D	Phenylalanine	F
Cysteine	C	Proline	P
Glutamic acid	E	Serine	S
Glutamine	Q	Threonine	T
Glycine	G	Tryptophan	W
Histidine	H	Tyrosine	Y
Isoleucine	I	Valine	V

not have the expected shape and consequently will not be able to function correctly.

4.3 GENETIC DAMAGE

Damage to DNA can be as a result of exposure to ionizing radiations, certain chemicals or viruses, and examples of each are given in *Table 4.3*. Chemicals that damage DNA are known as **mutagens** and if this causes cancer the chemical is called a **carcinogen**.

Table 4.3 Some causes of DNA damage

Physical	X-rays
	γ-rays
	Ultraviolet radiation
Chemical	Polycyclic aromatic hydrocarbons
	Asbestos
	Azo dyes
Viral	Epstein–Barr virus
	Human T-lymphotropic virus I
	Papillomavirus

Ionizing radiation

Ionizing radiation includes α and β radiation, protons and neutrons; electromagnetic radiation includes X-rays, γ-rays and ultraviolet radiation. These damage DNA directly either by breaking the strands or by forming pyrimidine dimers. Radiation also interacts with other molecules within the cell, often water, causing ionization and the formation of highly reactive free radicals which attack and damage DNA. Some tissues such as the bone marrow or the thyroid are more susceptible to radiation damage and tumour formation, and children are more susceptible than adults. This may be a reflection of the number of cells actively dividing in a given tissue or individual.

Mutagens and carcinogens

Some chemicals react directly with DNA in the cell, causing mutation of the base pair sequence. These chemicals tend to be highly reactive, forming covalent bonds with DNA and causing the formation of DNA adducts; examples of these include nitrogen mustards, benzyl chloride and bis-(chloromethyl) ether. Other chemicals are inactive but may become carcinogens by the action of particular enzymes; these chemicals are known as procarcinogens. The enzymes responsible for the conversion of a procarcinogen to an active carcinogen are the P_{450} enzymes. These are a highly polymorphic system of enzymes, with different individuals having different combinations of enzymes. This leads to some individuals being more susceptible to the formation of cancer because they have the particular P_{450} enzyme that transforms a procarcinogen to a carcinogen. Examples of compounds that are procarcinogens include polycyclic aromatic hydrocarbons found in cigarette smoke and in barbecued food. Aflatoxins, a natural product of a fungus, and vinyl chloride are further examples.

Viruses

There are two ways in which viruses alter host DNA. The first is by inserting their viral genome into host DNA at particular sites, causing activation and expression of the gene or gene modification. The second way is by expressing viral genes in the cell which transform the cell into a cancer cell (see *Box 4.3).*

Box 4.3 Rous sarcoma virus

In 1911, Francis Peyton Rous showed that a spontaneous tumour could be transplanted by cell grafts and cell-free extracts of the tumour. This indicated that a virus was responsible for causing the tumour. This famous example was Rous sarcoma virus. Several other animal tumours were shown to be of viral origin by the 1930s. Rous was awarded a Nobel Prize in 1966. In the late 1970s Michael Bishop and Harold Varmus first identified the presence of oncogenes in cells, for which they were awarded a Nobel Prize in 1989.

When DNA is damaged by ionizing radiation or a chemical carcinogen, a point mutation can occur, that is, a single nucleotide base is altered or deleted. Viruses can remove host DNA or insert new DNA into host DNA, and can switch on genes inappropriately, all of which can disrupt the normal function of the cell.

DNA has many repair mechanisms to prevent damaged DNA from being passed to the next generation of cells, and the body has other defence systems to prevent damage to DNA; examples are the production of anti-oxidants and detoxification of carcinogens by enzymes. Often the immune system can recognize cells that contain damaged DNA or viruses and destroy them. Occasionally the mutation is not detected or the repair mechanisms are not effective and the mutated gene will persist. Most mutations are never recognized because the damaged DNA is not involved in producing an important protein or the part of a protein that is important in interacting with other molecules.

If damage occurs to a reproductive cell, the damaged DNA can be passed to future generations of individuals. A damaged gene could be passed from generation to generation without ill-effect if an individual inherits a 'good' gene from the other parent and produces sufficient 'good' protein. In the unfortunate circumstance when a defective gene is inherited from both parents, there is no compensation by a good gene and the affected individual will develop a genetic disease. This is the subject of Chapter 11, where it is studied in greater depth and examples of such diseases are given.

If the damaged gene expresses an important protein, in other words it is important for the normal functioning of the cell, the protein produced will have a different amino acid sequence and consequently an abnormal function. If the gene is in a germ line cell and happens to code for an enzyme which is then inactive or has reduced activity to its substrate, then this could lead to an **inborn error of metabolism** (Chapter 11) in the next generation.

Damage to DNA in somatic cells, i.e. non-reproductive cells, can lead to the formation of cancer. If the damaged gene is involved in the regulation of cell growth and cell division, there is a loss of normal control that can result in tumour formation.

4.4 CANCER AND TUMOUR MARKERS

Damaged genes associated with cell growth and division are called **oncogenes** and are important in the formation of cancer. In health the normal gene is known as a **proto-oncogene**. Oncogenes drive the cell into continued, uncontrolled cell division. On the other hand, **tumour suppressor genes** arrest the cell growth cycle if there is damaged DNA, allowing the opportunity for repair of DNA. If the tumour suppressor gene is damaged and the gene product does not function, the cell cycle will not be halted and damaged DNA will not be repaired, allowing the passage of this mutated DNA to the next generation of cells. The damaged tumour suppressor gene is often known as an **anti-oncogene**.

Cancer is the uncontrolled growth of a single cell in which the normal control mechanisms have become defective due to damage of the growth control genes. The cell and its progeny continue to divide out of control, leading to the formation of a tumour. Tumour cells are often unstable and undergo further changes and some tumours can start to produce chemicals or proteins that the cell would not normally produce. These chemicals and proteins are expressed on the cell surface or released into the surrounding tissue fluids, and can then be detected in the blood and are known as **tumour markers**. Tumour markers can be chemicals that the cell does not normally make; for example, patients with cancer of the colon often produce carcinoembryonic antigen, not normally produced in adult life. If a cell normally synthesizes and secretes a chemical, a tumour of that cell could cause the uncontrolled production of that substance. This would lead to high levels in the blood; for example, in multiple myeloma, which is a cancer of antibody-producing cells, abnormal quantities of a single antibody are produced, causing the disease. Many endocrine diseases are caused by tumours of hormone-secreting cells that are not subject to normal control mechanisms, leading to abnormally high hormone levels in the blood. See the following chapters for more details of endocrine diseases.

In the clinical laboratory, much effort is taken in the detection of cancer by measuring levels of tumour markers and hormones. These measurements can be used to diagnose the disease, after the onset of symptoms, and then to monitor therapy. If the tumour is treated successfully, levels of the marker fall to within the reference range. If the tumour returns, the levels rise. A good example of this is the measurement of prostate-specific antigen (PSA), which is used to diagnose and monitor the treatment of prostate cancer. Further discussion of tumour markers is given in Chapter 12.

In recent years much new work has been centred on the detection of oncogenes, tumour suppressor genes and their protein products. *Table 4.4*

Table 4.4 Some important oncogenes, tumour suppressor genes and associated cancers

Oncogenes	
ABL/BCR	Chronic myeloid leukaemia
ErbB	Bladder and breast cancer
FOS	Osteosarcoma
HER2	Breast, stomach, ovarian and bladder cancers
JUN	Lung cancers
KIT	Lung cancer and acute myeloblastic leukaemia
MYC	Lung, breast and cervical cancers
RAS	Many, especially pancreatic and colon cancers
SRC	Colon, skin and breast cancers
TRK	Colon and thyroid cancers
Tumour suppressor genes	
BRCA1 and *2*	Breast cancer
DCC	Colon and ovarian cancers
p53	Most cancers
RB1	Retinoblastoma and many other cancers, especially lung, bladder and pancreatic

lists some of the more clinically useful oncogenes and suppressor genes that have been studied in the investigation of cancer.

4.5 GENETIC DISEASE AND THE CLINICAL BIOCHEMISTRY LABORATORY

Many modern clinical biochemistry laboratories now perform a range of techniques that look for defects in a specific gene or sequence of DNA. This application of molecular biology has led to the development of a new generation of diagnostic and screening tests being developed. One of the most powerful tests is the **polymerase chain reaction** (PCR). PCR is a highly sensitive technique that can, in theory, detect a single gene from just one strand of DNA. This high sensitivity is achieved by copying a preselected segment of the original DNA many thousands of times. Only the preselected DNA sequence is copied, so the assay can be designed to look for mutations in a particular part of a gene. *Figure 4.3* outlines the principle of the PCR technique. Obviously the sequence of the normal gene and mutated gene have to be known before a PCR method can be developed. Not so many years ago PCR was an involved technique, often taking many hours, but PCR is now automated and answers are available in 15–30 minutes (see *Box 4.4*).

Applications of PCR in clinical biochemistry include:

■ Diagnosis of inborn errors of metabolism;
■ Screening for cancer;
■ Prenatal diagnosis of genetic disease;
■ Detection of bacterial and viral infections.

Using PCR, many inherited diseases can be rapidly screened for and diagnosed, allowing appropriate action to be taken. Unfortunately, there is no cure for many genetic diseases, so treatment can only be palliative. One contentious use of PCR is prenatal screening for genetic disease in the foetus. The parents are given the opportunity of having the pregnancy terminated if a positive result is found. Usually these tests are only offered to parents who are at risk of having an affected child. Chapter 11 looks in more detail at the range of inborn errors of metabolism that are investigated in the clinical laboratory.

Genomics is the study of the entire genome, and saw a rapid expansion in the late 1990s. The related field of **proteomics** is the study of the complete expression of proteins in particular cells. New technology has developed **gene chips**, also known as microarrays, which can analyse many hundreds

Box 4.4 PCR

The polymerase chain reaction was devised by Kary Mullis, during a three-hour night drive in 1983. It took him only a year to test and improve the method that has become one of the most widely used techniques in modern molecular biology. He received a Nobel Prize for his work in 1993.

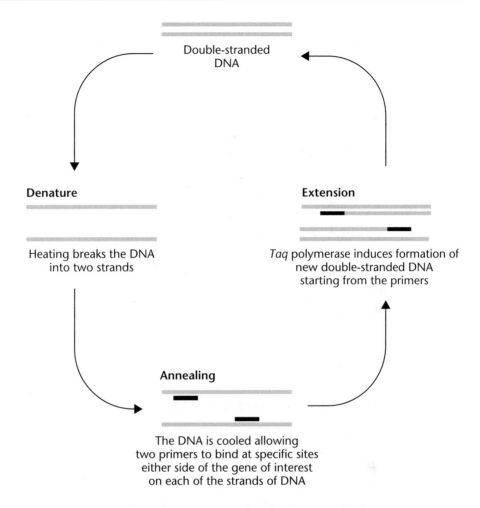

Figure 4.3
The polymerase chain reaction involves repeated cycles of denaturing double-stranded DNA by heating and cooling the DNA to allow two primers to anneal to the single strands of DNA, and allowing *Taq* DNA polymerase to extend the primers, forming new double-stranded DNA. The primers are carefully designed so they bind either side of the gene of interest. Each cycle doubles the number of target genes and, after a couple of cycles, it is only the gene sequence between the primers that is being copied. Thus, 25 cycles would yield 2^{25} copies of the gene, i.e. 33 554 432 copies.

or even thousands of genes in a single assay. These specialized tests use a microarray of DNA sequences which are immobilized on to a surface such as a glass slide. This technology is powerful for identifying DNA mutations and the expression of genes in diseases such as cancers and inborn errors of metabolism. These are just starting to be used in the routine diagnosis of disease, and genomics and proteomics can be expected to lead to the identification of new markers of disease which will be introduced into the routine laboratory as part of routine blood testing. In the future, microarrays may be used to screen every newborn baby to identifying genes which are associated with risk of future disease (see *Box 4.5*).

Box 4.5 Human Genome Project

The Human Genome Project was completed in 2003 and published all the individual chromosome structures by 2006. The project decoded more than three billion nucleotides and identified approximately 30 000 genes, which is fewer than was predicted.

SUGGESTED FURTHER READING

In addition to relevant chapters in the text books cited in Chapter 1 the following references are recommended.

Buckingham L. and Flaws M.L. (2007) *Molecular Diagnostics: Fundamentals, Methods and Clinical Applications*. Philadelphia: F.A. Davis.

Tsongalisa G.J. and Silverman L.M. (2006) Molecular diagnostics: a historical perspective. *Clinica Chimica Acta*, **369**: 188–192.

Read A.P. and Donnai D. (2007) *New Clinical Genetics*. Oxford, Scion Publishing.

Nakamura R.M. and Grody W. (2004) *Cancer Diagnostics: Current and Future Trends*. Totowa, NJ: Humana Press Inc.

Lodish H. and Darnell J.E. (2003) Molecular Cell Biology, 5th edition. New York: W.H. Freeman & Co Ltd.

SELF-ASSESSMENT QUESTIONS

1. Which bases pair with each other when two strands of DNA bind?
2. What is the name given to a triplet of nucleotides?
3. Which triplet can act as a start signal?
4. In a given gene, what is the name given to the DNA which is expressed in order to make proteins?
5. Why does mutated DNA cause a problem in cells?
6. What are damaged genes that cause cancer called?
7. What type of cancer-forming gene is p53?
8. What is the name of the powerful technique that can amplify a specific region of DNA?

Endocrinology – chemical control

Learning objectives
After studying this chapter you should confidently be able to:

■ **Explain how hormones exert their control on the body.**
Hormones act on other tissues distant from where they were synthesized.
Hormones travel in the blood stream, often bound to a carrier protein. It
is free hormone that is metabolically active.
Hormones bind to cell receptors in order to exert their action on a cell.
Hormone receptors are found on the cell surface and within the cell
(intracellular receptors) and steroid and thyroid hormones bind to
intracellular receptors. The level of hormone in blood is controlled by a
negative feedback loop.

■ **Describe the role of the hypothalamus and pituitary gland.**
The hypothalamus produces 'releasing' hormones that stimulate the
pituitary. The pituitary produces 'stimulating' hormones that cause
production of other hormones in other tissues.

■ **Broadly classify different types of endocrine disease.**
Endocrine disease can manifest as either hypofunction or hyperfunction of
an endocrine organ. Primary disease is one that affects the hormone-
producing tissue. Secondary disease is when the primary hormone-
producing tissue is inappropriately stimulated or suppressed by another
hormone. An ectopic hormone is a hormone or hormone-like substance
produced by a non-endocrine tumour.

■ **Give examples of dynamic function tests and explain why they are
used in the investigation of endocrine disease.**
Hormones are influenced by external factors such as stress and often have
to be diagnosed using a dynamic function test. Stimulation tests are
generally used to investigate hypofunction and suppression tests are
generally used to investigate hyperfunction.

■ **Describe the mechanism of an immunoassay used to measure a
hormone.**
Most hormones are measured by an immunoassay. Small molecules are
measured using competitive immunoassays. Large molecules are measured
using non-competitive immunoassays. A lateral flow immunoassay is the
basis of most pregnancy tests.

In the last chapter we saw how all the information required to control the normal function of the cells, that together make an individual, is stored in the DNA. In this and the subsequent chapters of this section we shall see how the 'day to day' metabolic control of many cells is regulated by the chemical messengers, called hormones. The system that produces and controls the production of hormones is called the endocrine system. Many cells produce and release chemical messengers that act on another cell, or sometimes the same cell (see *Fig. 5.1*). The definition of a hormone (the endocrine signal) is a chemical messenger that is synthesized and released by cells in one tissue and transported in the blood to exert its metabolic control on cells in another part of the body (see *Box 5.1*).

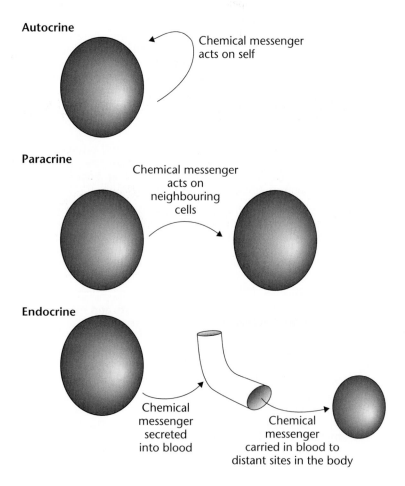

Autocrine

Chemical messenger acts on self

Paracrine

Chemical messenger acts on neighbouring cells

Endocrine

Chemical messenger secreted into blood

Chemical messenger carried in blood to distant sites in the body

Figure 5.1
The three types of interaction between cells and chemical messengers. Acting on self = autocrine; acting on a close neighbour = paracrine.; acting on cells at a distance, being carried in the blood stream = endocrine.

Box 5.1 Hormones

Jokichi Takamine (1854–1922), a Japanese–American biochemist, was the first to isolate a hormone (Ernest Starling coined the name hormone). In 1901 he was working on adrenal glands and extracted adrenaline in a crystalline form, the first pure hormone to be isolated from its natural tissue.

There are many endocrine organs in the body producing many different hormones. New hormones are being discovered every year. *Table 5.1* lists the major endocrine organs and the more important hormones.

Table 5.1 The major endocrine organs and important hormones produced by them

Organ	Hormone	Abbreviation
Hypothalamus	Corticotrophin-releasing hormone	CRH
	Gonadotrophin-releasing hormone	GnRH
	Thyrotrophin-releasing hormone	TRH
	Prolactin release-inhibiting hormone	PIH
	Growth hormone-releasing hormone	GRH
Pituitary (anterior)	Adrenocorticotrophic hormone	ACTH
	Thyroid-stimulating hormone	TSH
	Growth hormone	GH
	Prolactin	PRL
	Luteinizing hormone	LH
	Follicle-stimulating hormone	FSH
Pituitary (posterior)	Oxytocin	
	Vasopressin (antidiuretic hormone)	ADH
Thyroid	Thyroxine	T4
	Triiodothyronine	T3
	Calcitonin	
Parathyroid	Parathyroid hormone	PTH
Adrenal cortex	Cortisol	
	Aldosterone	
Adrenal medulla	Adrenaline	
	Noradrenaline	
Pancreas	Insulin	
Ovaries	Oestradiol	
	Progesterone	
Testes	Testosterone	
	Inhibin	
Gut	Gastrin	
	Secretin	
	Cholecystokinin	
	Motilin	
	Vasoactive peptide	VIP
	Gastric-inhibiting peptide	GIP
Heart	Atrial natriuretic peptide	ANP

Hormones can be classified according to the type of molecule from which they are derived. These are:

- **Steroid hormones**, for example cortisol. These hormones are all derived from cholesterol.
- **Amino acid derivatives**, for example, thyroid hormones.
- **Peptides and proteins**. This is the largest group containing large proteins such as TSH and small peptides such as TRH, which is a tripeptide.

5.1 TRANSPORT OF HORMONES

Hormones are released by a tissue and transported in the blood to the target organ. The thyroid hormones and steroid hormones are carried by a number of specific transport proteins in the blood: thyroxine binds to a protein called thyroxine-binding globulin, testosterone binds to sex hormone-binding globulin. It is the free hormone that is metabolically active; the bound hormone can act as a reservoir. The bound and free hormone are in equilibrium and, as free hormone is used, more hormone dissociates from the carrier protein to become active and to replace the used free hormone.

5.2 ACTION OF HORMONES

Hormones act at the cellular level causing a change in the cell's metabolic processes by increasing or decreasing the rate of synthesis of various molecules within the cell. This is brought about by the interaction of the hormone with a specific receptor. Most hormones bind with a receptor found on the cell surface. When a hormone binds to its receptor a cascade of reactions takes place inside the cell, called the cell signalling pathway. This activates a particular gene, or group of genes, starting the manufacture of new protein, which influences the synthetic pathways in the cell. Only cells with a hormone receptor will respond to the hormone; for example, TSH binds to TSH receptors on the surface of thyroid cells, causing the cell to increase its production of thyroid hormone.

Thyroid hormones and steroid hormones can cross the lipid cell membrane and bind to intracellular receptors. When the hormone binds to its receptor in the cell nucleus, the receptor forms a dimer, and this then binds directly to particular sequences of DNA, allowing activation of gene transcription.

5.3 CONTROL OF HORMONE PRODUCTION

Release of hormone from the hormone-producing cells is controlled by a negative feedback loop. High levels of hormone result in the reduction of its synthesis and release into the blood. Conversely, low levels of hormone induce its synthesis via the negative feedback loop. *Figure 5.2* shows the

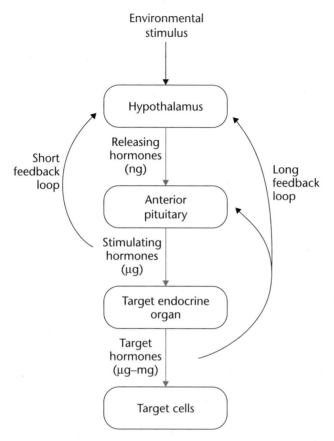

Figure 5.2
The negative feedback loops of the hypothalamic–pituitary axis (refer to text for details).

negative feedback loops for the hypothalamic–pituitary axis. The concentration of hormone from the target organ acts on receptors in the hypothalamus and the pituitary gland, regulating the release of the stimulating hormones that act on the target organ.

Hypothalamic hormones are also under the control of neural stimuli that may override other control mechanisms. Stress and mental illness may give rise to the abnormal hormone levels found in endocrine disease. This reaction to stress can be used to test the endocrine pathway. Hypothalamic hormones show an episodic type of release and follow a regular secretory rhythm, where often the time of greatest release is around dawn whereas the time of lowest release is during the hours before midnight.

5.4 THE HYPOTHALAMIC–PITUITARY AXIS

The hypothalamic–pituitary axis (HPA) is a major endocrine pathway acting on a number of **target organs** and thereby regulating a large number of hormones. *Figure 5.2* shows the HPA and how it acts as an **amplification cascade**. The hypothalamus produces nanogram amounts of hormones called releasing factors which act on specific cells in the pituitary to release microgram quantities of stimulating hormone. This, in turn, results in milligram quantities of hormone being released from the target organ. The target organs affected by the HPA are the thyroid, adrenal gland and the gonads (Chapter 6 deals with thyroid hormones). Other pituitary hormones are less specific in their action and can act on many different cells and organs, for example growth hormone. The concentration of the final hormone from the target organ is controlled via the **negative feedback loop**. In this control loop, rising levels of hormone act on the hypothalamus and the pituitary to reduce the amount of releasing and stimulating hormones, thereby reducing the amount of the final hormone being released by the endocrine organ. Falling or low levels of hormone in the blood result in higher levels of releasing and stimulating hormones being released by the hypothalamus and pituitary, thereby having the effect of raising hormone production and release from the endocrine organ. The short negative feedback loop operates between the hormones released from the anterior pituitary and the hypothalamus, whereas the long negative feedback loop allows the hormone from the target endocrine organ to control the hypothalamus and pituitary.

The hypothalamus and pituitary are closely related. The hypothalamus is part of the brain, situated under the thalamus, and has many neural connections with other parts of the brain, which is why environmental and neurological factors can influence the endocrine system. The pituitary gland is a small pea-sized organ, weighing about half a gram, and attached to the hypothalamus by a short stalk. The gland is divided into two lobes: the **anterior pituitary** (adenohypophysis) and the **posterior pituitary** (neurohypophysis). The anterior pituitary is connected to the hypothalamus by a network of capillaries and is stimulated to release pituitary hormones in response to hypothalamic hormones released into these capillaries. Between the posterior pituitary and the hypothalamus, there are neural connections that transport hormones synthesized in the hypothalamus to the posterior pituitary for release into the blood. Despite its small size, the pituitary regulates many of the body's functions via the hormones it synthesizes and is sometimes known as the 'master endocrine gland'.

The important hormones released by the anterior pituitary are:

- **Thyroid-stimulating hormone** (TSH): released from the pituitary in response to the hypothalamic hormone thyrotrophin-releasing hormone (TRH). TSH acts on the follicle cells of the thyroid to bring about the release of thyroid hormones (see Chapter 6).
- **Adrenocorticotrophic hormone** (ACTH): released in response to corticotrophin-releasing hormone (CRH) and acts on the adrenal gland to increase the synthesis and release of cortisol.
- The gonadotrophins, **luteinizing hormone** (LH) and **follicle-stimulating hormone** (FSH): these are released from the pituitary in response to the hypothalamic hormone gonadotrophin-releasing

hormone (GnRH). LH acts on the Leydig cells of the testes to bring about the release of testosterone. In females LH acts on the corpus luteum in the ovary to cause the production and release of progesterone. FSH acts on the Sertoli cells in the testes to increase spermatogenesis and in the female, FSH causes the maturation of the ovum and the production of oestradiol (see *Box 5.2*).

■ **Prolactin** (PRL): acts on the mammary glands to stimulate the production of breast milk. The release of PRL is controlled by a positive feedback loop in response to suckling. In the absence of suckling, dopamine, produced by the hypothalamus, is thought to act as a prolactin release-inhibiting factor.

■ **Growth hormone** (GH): released in response to growth hormone-releasing hormone (GRH), also known as somatocrinin. GH acts on many cells to produce insulin-like growth factors and stimulate cell growth.

Box 5.2 Sex hormones

Adolf Butenandt, a German organic chemist, isolated pure oestrone from urine of pregnant women; the first purified sex hormone. Later he isolated 15 mg of androsterone from 15 000 litres of urine donated by Viennese policemen and 20 mg of progesterone from the ovaries of 50 000 sows. He was awarded a Nobel Prize for his work in 1939.

5.5 ENDOCRINE DISORDERS

To maintain health the body's metabolism needs to be controlled within fine limits that are achieved by the complex interaction of many hormones. If the production of a hormone is altered and the blood concentration becomes inappropriate, this leads to loss of control of part of the metabolism, resulting in an endocrine disorder and its associated clinical symptoms. In general, endocrine disease can be divided into two classes: an **inappropriate overproduction** of a hormone and the **inappropriate underproduction** of a hormone. In the HPA, disease which affects the target directly is called a primary disorder, leading to hypo- or hyperfunction of that organ, whilst disease of the hypothalamus or pituitary leads to a secondary disorder of the target tissue but the symptoms at clinical presentation are the same.

The inappropriate overproduction of a hormone, or **hyperfunction**, is often due to a tumour of a hormone-producing cell. Sometimes a tumour elsewhere in the body can produce a hormone or a hormone-like substance, referred to as an **ectopic hormone**. The hormone being produced by a tumour is not subject to the negative feedback control and so hormone is constantly being produced, causing an increase in blood concentration, even when the normal control mechanisms are trying to reduce the blood concentration. In primary disease the tumour is located in the target organ and normal negative feedback control operates which suppresses the production of the stimulatory hormones from the hypothalamus and pituitary. A hormone-producing tumour in the hypothalamus or the pituitary will drive the rest of the HPA, resulting in a secondary disorder of the target organ and causing the uncontrolled production of hormone from that organ. The normal feedback loop does not operate, as the high levels of hormone from the target organ do not suppress the formation of stimulatory hormone that is forcing the production of target hormone. The high levels of hormone from the target organ, whether due to a primary or secondary disease, result in a clinical picture associated with excess hormone production from the target organ. An example of this is a thyroid tumour and a pituitary adenoma producing TSH (driving the thyroid to produce thyroid hormones); both result in a clinical picture of hyperthyroidism.

The inappropriate underproduction of a hormone, or **hypofunction**, often results from destruction or malformation of hormone-producing tissue or cells. The destruction of tissue can be due to an infection, trauma, infiltration by a tumour, infarction or iatrogenic causes such as radiation treatment. Primary hypofunction of one of the target organs leads to reduced levels of circulating hormone from that organ and, through the normal negative feedback mechanisms, the hypothalamus and pituitary respond by increasing the synthesis and release of their hormones which are trying to increase production of the target organ hormone. Secondary disease caused by hypofunction of the hypothalamus or pituitary results in low levels of circulating target organ hormone. In this case, the negative feedback control does not function, as the low levels of target hormone do not stimulate the damaged hypothalamus or pituitary to produce their hormones. *Table 5.2* shows changes seen in the level of hypothalamic–pituitary–target organ axis hormones in primary, secondary and ectopic endocrine disease. Examples of different endocrine diseases and the hormones involved are given in *Table 5.3*.

Table 5.2 Changes seen in hormone levels of the hypothalamic–pituitary–target organ axis in endocrine disease

	Clinical picture	Pituitary hormone	Target organ hormone
Primary disease of the target organ	Hyperfunction	↓	↑
	Hypofunction	↑	↓
Secondary disease of the target organ	Hyperfunction	↑	↑
	Hypofunction	↓	↓
Ectopic hormone	Hyperfunction	↓	↑

Table 5.3 Important clinical conditions associated with pituitary hormones

Hormone	Hyperfunction	Hypofunction
TSH	Hyperthyroidism	Hypothyroidism
ACTH	Cushing's disease	Secondary adrenal hypofunction
LH/FSH	Precocious puberty	Secondary hypogonadism
PRL	Infertility Amenorrhoea	Failure of lactation
GH	Gigantism Acromegaly	Dwarfism

5.6 INVESTIGATION OF ENDOCRINE DISEASE

In the clinical biochemistry laboratory many hormones are measured, giving an indication of the concentration in the blood at the time the sample was taken. This is a 'snapshot' of a complex dynamic system of hormone regulation. In some circumstances a single hormone measurement may be sufficient to confirm a diagnosis; for example, a patient with classical hyperthyroidism will have an elevated thyroid hormone concentration (thyroid hormones are discussed fully in the next chapter). Sometimes further investigations are required to evaluate the hormone status of the patient. The concentration of some hormones, such as cortisol, can be influenced by external factors that cannot easily be controlled, for example stress. In these situations a **dynamic function** test may be performed. Dynamic function tests follow serial measurements of the hormone after the hormonal pathway has been stressed in some way. Three main types of dynamic function test can be defined: stimulation tests, suppression tests and stress tests.

Stimulation tests

These tests are designed to stimulate the release of a hormone, often using synthetic releasing or stimulatory hormones given by intravenous injection. Normally the target endocrine organ will respond by producing high levels of hormone, which are measured in blood samples taken at 0, 20, 60 and sometimes 120 minutes (see *Fig. 5.3a*). The 0 minute sample is taken just before the stimulatory hormone is given and represents the basal level. If there is primary endocrine disease, the target endocrine organ is unresponsive to stimulation and there is no increase in the concentration of measured hormone over the time the blood samples are taken. In the case of secondary endocrine disease, where the pituitary or hypothalamus is affected, stimulation can induce an increase in hormone released by the target endocrine organ over the time the blood samples are taken. A good example of this

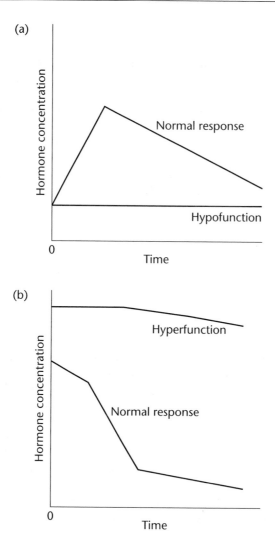

Figure 5.3
Responses to dynamic function tests. (a) A stimulation test: a normal response shows a rise in hormone concentration not seen in patients with hypofunction. (b) A supression test: a normal response shows a fall in hormone concentration not seen in patients with hyperfunction.

type of investigation is the Synacthen stimulation test. Synacthen is synthetic ACTH used in the investigation of adrenal hypofunction (Addison's disease). A normal response is an increase in cortisol following an intra-muscular injection of Synacthen, whereas no increase is seen in a patient with Addison's disease. Stimulation tests are useful in differentiating between primary and secondary hypofunction disease states.

Suppression tests

Suppression tests are designed to suppress or downregulate the hypothalamic–pituitary–target organ axis, often using a synthetic hormone. The test is performed in much the same way as for stimulation tests and the response of a hormone is measured over time, often over a number of days rather than minutes or hours. Suppression tests are usually employed to investigate hyperfunction disease states. A normal response to suppression is a drop in hormone concentration, whereas a failure to suppress, or only partial suppression, would indicate inappropriate hormone production (see *Fig. 5.3b*). An example of a widely used suppression test is the dexamethasone suppression test for investigating patients with high cortisol levels. Dexamethasone is a synthetic steroid that has the effect of suppressing ACTH production by the pituitary, thereby downregulating the HPA. Failure to suppress cortisol levels suggests an autonomous production of hormone by the adrenal gland or by an ectopic source of hormone located in another tissue such as the lungs.

Stress tests

These tests impose physiological stress on the body and the response by hormones is monitored. The most important test is the insulin stress test, where insulin is administered to the patient in order to induce hypoglycaemic stress. This test is used to investigate patients with high levels of cortisol who do not respond to the dexamethasone suppression test. Cortisol is a stress hormone and would normally rise as a response to insulin-induced hypoglycaemia, whereas a patient with Cushing's syndrome would not show a rise in blood cortisol concentration. The insulin stress test has also been used in the investigation of patients suspected of having GH deficiency. GH levels in blood increase in response to stress, and failure to demonstrate an increase in GH following an insulin stress test indicates an inappropriate underproduction.

5.7 MEASUREMENT OF HORMONES

Hormones are present in the blood at very low concentrations and particularly sensitive techniques are required to measure such low levels. Many very sensitive techniques, called immunoassays, have been developed for this purpose and rely on the use of the specific binding properties of antibodies. The concentration of any hormone can be measured by choosing an antibody (or pair of antibodies) that only binds to that hormone. Immunoassays also require a label attached to one of the components of the immunoassay system. Common labels used are radioisotopes, enzymes, and fluorescent and luminescent molecules; examples of each are given in *Table 5.4*. Labels used should be easily measured and not prone to interference.

Table 5.4 Common labels used in immunoassay techniques and method of detection

Type of label	Example	Detection
Radioisotopes	^{125}I, ^{14}C, ^{3}H	α-rays, β-particles
Enzymes	Alkaline phosphatase Horseradish peroxidase Malate dehydrogenase	Measurement of a coloured product from a substrate
Fluorescent	Fluorecein isothiocyanate Rhodamine Red Europium chelates	Photons of light
Luminescent	Luminol Acridinium esters	Photons of light

There are two main types of immunoassay, namely competitive and non-competitive assays (see *Box 5.3*).

Competitive immunoassay

This was the original type of assay developed in the early 1960s, also known as a competitive binding assay. The principle is that a constant amount of labelled antigen (Ag*) is added to an unknown amount of antigen (Ag) from the patient's sample and then mixed with a limited amount of antibody to that antigen, resulting in competition between the labelled and patient's antigen for the binding sites on the antibody. Many new techniques use an antibody that has been immobilized on to a solid surface rather than the antibody being in solution. Once the antibody/Ag reaction has taken place, unreacted label (**free** label) is removed, leaving only the reacted label (**bound** label) in the tube. The amount of label remaining in the tube is then measured. If there is a low concentration of antigen in the patient's sample then there will be a large number of binding sites on the antibody which bind to labelled antigen. Conversely, a high concentration of antigen in the patient's sample will result in a low number of antibody binding sites which contain labelled antigen. The classic competitive assay dose–response curve is shown in *Fig. 5.4*.

Competitive assays are usually used for small antigens such as the thyroid hormones which have only a single binding site (an epitope), and are usually not as sensitive as non-competitive assays. Examples of competitive assays

---

Box 5.3 Development of the first radioimmunoassay

Rosalyn Yalow and her colleague S. A. Berson developed the first radioimmunoassay in the late 1950s. She was awarded a Nobel Prize for her work in 1977.

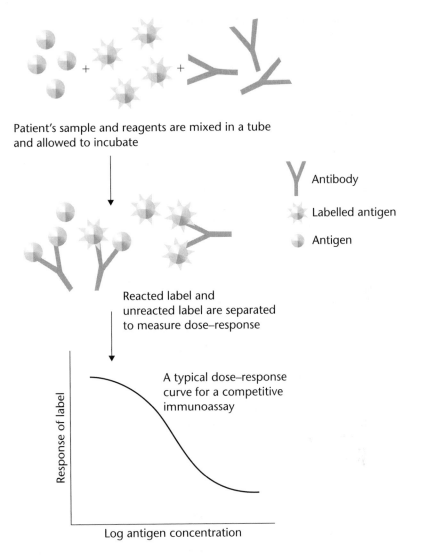

Patient's sample and reagents are mixed in a tube and allowed to incubate

Antibody

Labelled antigen

Antigen

Reacted label and unreacted label are separated to measure dose–response

A typical dose–response curve for a competitive immunoassay

Response of label

Log antigen concentration

Figure 5.4
The stages of a competitive immunoassay and the typical dose–response curve.

commonly used in a clinical biochemistry laboratory are radioimmuno-assay (RIA), enzyme-multiplied immunoassay technique (EMIT) and polar-ized fluorescent immunoassay.

Non-competitive immunoassay (sandwich assay)

This type of assay generally uses an antibody which has been immobilized on a solid phase such as the inside of a test tube, a microtitre plate well or the surface of a polystyrene bead. The immobilized antibody captures antigen from the patient's sample, causing the antigen to be bound by the 'capture antibody' to the solid phase. A wash step at this stage removes unreacted sample and any potential interference. A second, labelled antibody is now added and allowed to react with the antigen, forming a sandwich on the solid phase. Unreacted, labelled antibody is removed by another washing step and the remaining bound label is measured. The greater the concentration of antigen present in the patient's sample, the greater the amount of label detected, giving a dose–response curve with a positive slope, as shown in *Fig. 5.5*.

This type of assay will only work on larger molecules where there are at least two separate epitopes on the antigen, one for each of the antibodies

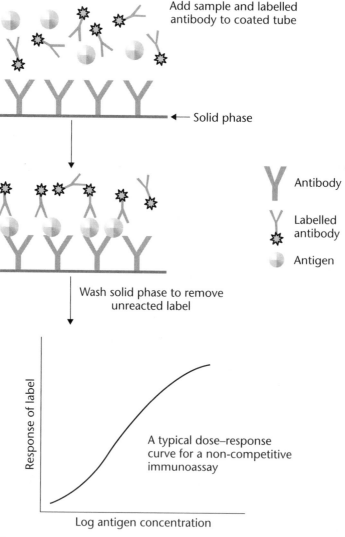

Figure 5.5
The stages of a non-competitive immunoassay and the typical dose–response curve.

used in the assay. Depending on the label used, this technique can be highly sensitive, detecting concentrations as low as 10^{-18} M. Fluorescent and luminescent labels are used in the most sensitive assays. Examples of non-competitive assays used in clinical biochemistry laboratories include enzyme-linked immunosorbent assay (ELISA), where an enzyme is the label used, and dissociation-enhanced lanthanide fluorescence immunoassay (DELFIA), which employs a europium label that becomes highly fluorescent in a special enhancing fluid.

Lateral flow immunoassay

An assay format first developed in the 1970s has revolutionized the way that immunoassays can be performed both rapidly and simply by unskilled operatives. These one-step tests are based on immunochromatographic techniques and are better known as lateral flow immunoassays. The principle is based on moving the sample through porous membranes by capillary action. Probably the most well-known example of a lateral flow immunoassay is the pregnancy test that can be bought over the counter in pharmacies. *Fig. 5.6* shows a diagram of a lateral flow immunoassay.

For larger molecules such as peptide hormones, the lateral flow immunoassay operates in a non-competitive or sandwich mode, with one antibody being immobilized on a porous membrane and the other antibody being immobilized on the surface of a particle. The particulate label is either a colloidal gold particle or a latex particle – this is also known as the conjugate. Gold particles are usually a red–purple colour, whereas latex can be fabricated in many different colours, most commonly blue. The analyte in

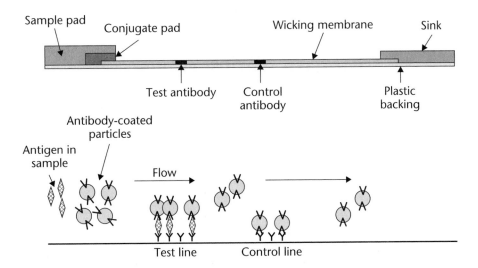

Figure 5.6
A lateral flow immunoassay device showing particles from a test line and control line (refer to text for details).

the sample binds to both antibodies and causes the particles to be captured on the wicking membrane, forming a visible line. There are two lines of antibody deposited on the membrane: one is specific to the analyte and the other is a control antibody. The labelled particles are dried in a special filter pad known as the conjugate pad. Also built into the device are a sample pad and a highly absorbent pad known as the sink, which pulls liquid through the membrane when the fluid reaches the end of the wicking membrane. Sample is added to the sample pad which then travels to the conjugate pad and rehydrates the labelled particles. The particles are moved through the membranes by capillary action, during which time the antibodies on the surface of the particle react with the antigen in the sample. Capillary action continues to pull liquid and particles through the wicking membrane and across the antibodies immobilized in a line at particular points. At the test line, the antigen in the sample, captured on the particle surface, will bind to the immobilized antibody on the membrane and cross-link the particle to the membrane, forming a coloured line visible to the eye. The control line has antibody immobilized on the membrane which will bind to the antibody on the particle, causing a line to be formed when antibody-coated particles are captured. When the assay is complete, particles will have moved through the wicking membrane by capillary action, passing across the test and control antibodies; a positive result is indicated by two visible lines on the membrane, one for the test and one for the control. A negative result is indicated by only the control line being visible.

A lateral flow immunoassay is ideal for situations where a 'yes/no' answer is required, such as a pregnancy test. New technology is being developed which is able to quantify the intensity of the line, by measuring the intensity of the colour. This will give rise to rapid, sensitive assays which do not require any instrumentation, for a range of hormones and other proteins. For small molecules, lateral flow assays have been developed that work on a competitive format.

SUGGESTED FURTHER READING

In addition to relevant chapters in the text books cited in Chapter 1 the following references are recommended.

Brook C. and Marshall N.J. (2001) *Essential Endocrinology*, 4th edition. Oxford: Blackwell Science Ltd.

Kronenberg H.M., Melmed S., Polonsky K.S. and Larsen P.R. (2007) *Williams' Textbook of Endocrinology*, 11th edition. Philadelphia: W.B. Saunders.

Lepage R. and Albert C. (2006) Fifty years of development in the endocrinology laboratory. *Clinical Biochemistry*, **39**: 542–557.

Malabanan A.O., Meikle A.W. and Swenson L. (2004) *Choose the Right Tests: Endocrine Disorders: The Primary Care Guide to Diagnostic Training*. Columbus, OH: Anadem Publishing.

Wild D. (2004) *The Immunoassay Handbook*, 3rd edition. Oxford: Elsevier.

Wong R. (2008) *Lateral Flow Immunoassay*. Totowa, NJ: Humana Press Inc.

SELF-ASSESSMENT QUESTIONS

1. Which hormones are produced by the thyroid gland?
2. What sort of molecule is cortisol?
3. In what form is a metabolically active hormone?
4. How do hormones exert their action on a cell?
5. What mechanism controls the level of hormone in the blood?
6. Which organ is sometimes known as the 'master endocrine gland'?
7. What are the two major types of endocrine disorder?
8. In primary hyperthyroidism, would you expect a raised or lowered TSH?
9. What sort of dynamic test would you use to investigate hypofunction disease?
10. For what sort of compound would a non-competitive immunoassay not be useful?

Thyroid hormones

Learning objectives
After studying this chapter you should confidently be able to:

■ **Describe the hormones of the hypothalamic–pituitary–thyroid axis.**
The synthesis and release of thyroid hormones is controlled by TSH, released from the pituitary gland and TRH, released from the hypothalamus. The two thyroid hormones produced by the thyroid are thyroxine (T_4) and triiodothyronine (T_3). Most of the thyroid hormone in blood is bound to transport proteins. The major transport proteins are thyroid-binding globulin, pre-albumin and albumin. It is the free hormone fraction that is physiologically active. A negative feedback loop controls levels of thyroid hormone in the blood.

■ **Describe the changes in the concentration of thyroid hormones found in different thyroid diseases and give examples of common thyroid disorders.**
Hyperthyroidism is the overproduction of thyroid hormones. Hypothyroidism is the underproduction of thyroid hormones. Primary disease is of the thyroid gland, secondary disease is of the pituitary or even hypothalamus. Graves' disease results from autoantibody stimulation of TSH receptors on the thyroid. All newborn infants are screened for congenital hypothyroidism.

■ **Describe laboratory methods used to measure thyroid hormones.**
Thyroid hormones are measured using immunoassays. Most modern laboratories measure free thyroid hormones. Most thyroid pathology can be diagnosed using ultrasensitive TSH measurements and free thyroid hormone measurements.

In the previous chapter we saw how the hypothalamic–pituitary axis controls the production and release of target organ hormones. This chapter will concentrate on the investigation and evaluation of a single target organ: the thyroid. The hypothalamic–pituitary–thyroid axis (HPTA) is a model for the other hormonal control systems, namely control of glucocorticoid hormones made in the adrenal cortex, and the gonadal hormones. The rationale behind the investigation of thyroid disease can be transferred to the investigation of endocrine disorders involving cortisol or the sex hormones.

Thyroid diseases result when the control mechanisms which keep the thyroid hormones within physiological limits are impaired or lost. The hormones are synthesized within the thyroid gland under the control of thyroid-stimulating hormone from the anterior pituitary, which in turn is controlled by thyrotropic-releasing hormone from the hypothalamus (see *Box 6.1*).

Box 6.1 Isolation of thyroxine

Edward Kendall (1886–1972) was an American biochemist who isolated thyroxine from thyroid tissue. He also studied the hormones of the adrenal cortex and isolated a series of steroids in the 1930s. He went on to discover cortisone and later won a Nobel Prize for his work on corticosteroids.

6.1 THE THYROID GLAND

The thyroid is a small, butterfly-shaped gland found at the base of the neck, in front and either side of the trachea. It has two lobes, each approximately 2×4 cm, joined by a thin piece of tissue called the isthmus. The secretion units of the gland contain follicles that contain colloid and are surrounded by a layer of epithelial cells. The colloid is mainly **thyroglobulin**, which has an important role to play in the synthesis of the thyroid hormones. Between the follicles are a number of cells called the C-cells that produce calcitonin.

In a number of conditions the thyroid becomes enlarged, a condition called **goitre**. Goitre can develop if the thyroid is overactive (hyperthyroidism) or underactive (hypothyroidism). Sometimes goitre develops when normal levels of hormone are present in the blood. Biochemical analysis of the blood will show which type of thyroid disease is causing the enlarged thyroid gland.

6.2 THYROID HORMONES

The thyroid synthesizes two thyroid hormones, **thyroxine** (3,5,3′,5′-L-tetraiodothyronine) and **triiodothyronine** (3,5,3′-L-triiodothyronine), commonly known as T_4 and T_3, respectively. These are synthesized by combining two iodinated tyrosyl residues on the surface of **thyroglobulin** in the thyroid follicles. Iodine is required in the diet to iodinate these tyrosyl residues and a lack of iodine results in diminished amounts of thyroid hormone being synthesized. The structures of T_4 and T_3 are shown in *Fig. 6.1*.

The thyroid hormones are released from the surface of the thyroglobulin when a follicular cell engulfs and digests particles of thyroglobulin from the follicles and releases T_4 and T_3 into the blood. T_4 is the main hormone produced and secreted by the thyroid. In the blood T_4 and T_3 rapidly bind to **transport proteins**, the three most important being **thyroid-binding**

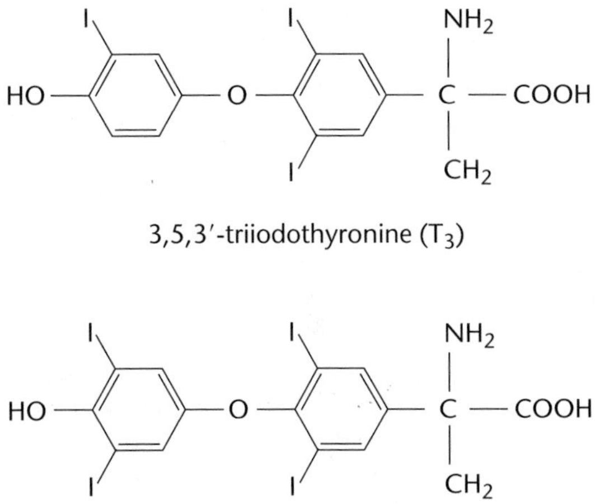

3,5,3'-triiodothyronine (T$_3$)

3,5,3',5'-tetraiodothyronine (T$_4$)

Figure 6.1
Structure of the two main thyroid hormones.

globulin (TBG), **pre-albumin** and **albumin**. The binding capacity of the proteins for thyroid hormones is usually only one-third saturated, and this means that 99.9% of thyroid hormones are bound to the transport proteins in blood. It is only the very tiny fraction of hormone that is not bound to the transport proteins, the **free hormone**, which is physiologically active.

6.3 ACTION OF THYROID HORMONES

Although T$_4$ is the major thyroid hormone present in the blood, it is T$_3$ that is the active hormone at the cellular level. In the cells that are sensitive to thyroid hormones, T$_4$ is converted by the process of deiodination into T$_3$. This suggests that T$_4$ is acting as a prehormone that is always available and can provide a source of T$_3$ at short notice. Inside the cell T$_3$ binds to hormone receptors in the nucleus, causing an increase in energy expenditure indicated by increased oxygen consumption. In the body thyroid hormones have important roles in:

- Growth;
- Sexual maturation;
- Development of the body;
- Increasing protein synthesis;
- Stimulating carbohydrate metabolism;
- Increasing lipid turnover;
- Maintenance of body weight.

6.4   **THYROID HORMONE HOMEOSTASIS**

The thyroid hormones are synthesized and released from the thyroid under the control of hormones released by the hypothalamic–pituitary axis (HPA). The hypothalamus synthesizes and releases thyrotropic-releasing hormone (TRH), a tripeptide. TRH acts on cells in the pituitary gland via TRH receptors, to produce and release **thyroid-stimulating hormone** (TSH) which binds to TSH receptors on cells within the thyroid gland, stimulating the synthesis and release of T_4 and T_3. TSH is a large glycoprotein with a molecular weight of 30 kDa and is composed of two subunits called α and β.

A negative feedback loop regulates the thyroid hormone concentration in the blood within tight limits. Rising levels of the thyroid hormones cause the pituitary not to respond to TRH, thereby reducing TSH production. Also, the action of thyroid hormones on cells within the hypothalamus reduces the production and release of TRH. Falling levels of thyroid

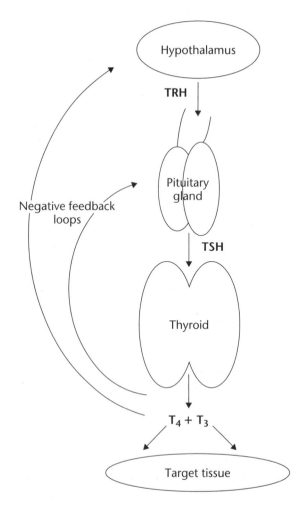

Figure 6.2
Hormones involved in the hypothalamic–pituitary–thyroid axis and the negative feedback loops.

hormones in the blood cause TRH and TSH secretion to be increased. *Figure 6.2* shows the HPTA and the associated negative feedback loops. In health, total T_4 is maintained in the range 65–130 nmol l^{-1} and total T_3 in the range 1.85–3.00 nmol l^{-1}. As mentioned previously, it is the free hormone that is physiologically active and exerts feedback control.

6.5 THYROID DISEASE

As with any endocrine disease there are two major categories of thyroid disease: **hypothyroidism** – a low blood thyroid hormone concentration, and **hyperthyroidism** – a high blood thyroid hormone concentration. Thyroid disease is investigated using **thyroid function tests**, which traditionally measured the concentration of total T_4. More recently, this has been replaced by measuring the concentration of the free hormones (FT_4 and FT_3) and TSH. The free hormone measurements have the advantage of not being affected by abnormal levels of binding proteins. In conditions where the binding proteins are unusually high or low, the total hormone levels reflect these changes and could be misinterpreted. For example, in the rare disorder of TBG deficiency, where there is an absence of TBG, the total T_4 is very low although the FT_4 is normal. Conversely, in pregnancy the production of transport proteins is increased, including TBG, causing the total T_4 to be raised, but FT_4 is normal.

Another development that has influenced the investigation of thyroid disease is the introduction of newer, ultrasensitive methods for measuring very low amounts of hormones such as TSH. In most modern laboratories a combination of TSH as a 'front-line' test and FT_4 or FT_3 is used. The exact combination of tests depends on the particular laboratory.

Hyperthyroidism

Hyperthyroidism is the inappropriate production of thyroid hormones resulting in blood concentrations of total and free hormone above the reference range. This is also called **thyrotoxicosis**. There are many causes of hyperthyroidism, which is often diagnosed by the clinical picture; blood tests confirm the diagnosis and help to identify the cause. The symptoms of hyperthyroidism include:

- Weight loss;
- Tachycardia;
- Agitation;
- Muscle weakness and tremor;
- Sweating and heat intolerance;
- Diarrhoea;
- Goitre;
- Exophthalmos (see *Box 6.2*).

The causes of hyperthyroidism can be classified into primary and secondary causes. Primary hyperthyroidism is the most commonly seen, and

Box 6.2 Exophthalmos

Exophthalmos is the accumulation of adipose tissue behind the eye, pushing the eye forward. This results in the patient having bulging eyes. This is a common sign of hyperthyroidism.

is due to a problem in the thyroid gland allowing excessive production and secretion of thyroid hormones. In these cases TSH levels are suppressed, often to undetectable levels, as a result of negative feedback on the pituitary and hypothalamus by high levels of T_4 and T_3. The most common causes of hyperthyroidism are:

- Graves' disease;
- Toxic multinodular goitre;
- Solitary toxic adenoma;
- Thyroiditis;
- Excessive T_4 and T_3 intake.

Of these, the most common cause of hyperthyroidism is **Graves' disease**, which is an autoimmune condition caused by the body's immune system producing antibodies against its own tissues; these are known as **autoantibodies**. The autoantibodies bind to TSH receptors in the thyroid, simulating the action of TSH and thus stimulating the production of T_4 and T_3. As there is not a control mechanism to prevent the autoantibodies binding to the receptors, there is continual stimulation of the thyroid gland, leading to goitre. In other cases, small tumours in the thyroid gland called adenomas can secrete thyroxine autonomously, i.e. without being influenced by the normal control mechanisms. The tumours are called 'toxic' as they cause the patient to become **thyrotoxic**, i.e. the patient suffers from the effects of too much thyroxine. These tumours may be solitary or multinodular. Primary hyperthyroidism is characterized by high T_4 and low TSH levels.

In some patients with symptoms of thyrotoxicosis the T_4 level is normal with a suppressed TSH, but T_3 is elevated. This condition is known as **T_3 toxicosis**. Rarer still is secondary hyperthyroidism, which is caused by a tumour in the pituitary secreting TSH, which in turn drives the thyroid. The tumour cells do not respond to normal control mechanisms, resulting in the autonomous production of TSH. Secondary hyperthyroidism is characterized by high T_4 levels with an elevated TSH.

Hypothyroidism

Hypothyroidism is the inappropriate underproduction of T_4 and T_3, resulting in concentrations of hormone in the blood below the reference range. The most likely cause is failure of the thyroid; so-called primary hypothyroidism. The following symptoms are associated with hypothyroidism:

- Weight gain;
- Cold intolerance;
- Lethargy and tiredness;

- Coarse hair and dry skin;
- Slow reflexes;
- Hoarseness;
- Anaemia.

As before, the causes can be classified into primary and secondary causes. Primary causes are associated with failure of the thyroid gland and consequent loss in production of the thyroid hormones. The causes of hypothyroidism include:

- Hashimoto's disease;
- Treatment of hyperthyroidism;
- TSH deficiency (secondary hypothyroidism);
- Iodine deficiency.

Of these, one of the commonest causes of hypothyroidism is the autoimmune disease known as **Hashimoto's disease**, which is an autoimmune disease where autoantibodies lead to the destruction of the thyroid gland and therefore loss of hormone synthesis. One other common cause is the treatment of hyperthyroid conditions by surgery or by radioactive iodine, leaving the patient unable to synthesize sufficient amounts of thyroid hormone and thereby resulting in hypothroidism. In response to the low thyroid hormone levels, the negative feedback control on the pituitary gland stimulates the production of TSH, elevating the blood concentration in an effort to drive the thyroid to produce more thyroxine. Primary hypothyroidism is characterized by a low T_4 and a high TSH.

Rarely, the symptoms suffered by the patient are due to secondary hypothyroidism, caused by damage to the HPA. In this condition, which can result from a head injury or a tumour of the pituitary gland, there is an inability to produce enough TSH to maintain concentrations of thyroxine within the reference range. Secondary hypothyroidism is characterized by low T_4 and low TSH levels. *Table 6.1* summarizes changes seen in hormone levels in the different thyroid conditions.

Table 6.1 Hormone changes associated with thyroid disease

Thyroid condition	T_4	T_3	TSH
Primary hyperthyroidism	↑	↑	↓
Secondary hyperthyroidism	↑	↑	↑
T_3 toxicosis	N	↑	↓
Primary hypothyroidism	↓	↓	↑
Secondary hypothyroidism	↓	↓	↓

N, Normal levels.

Congenital hypothyroidism

This is a condition that may be due to defects in making thyroid hormones or due to an absence of the thyroid gland (athyreosis). This occurs in approximately 1 in 4000 live births. The lack of thyroxine causes failure to thrive and severe mental impairment, called cretinism. If diagnosed soon after birth, thyroxine can be given, allowing normal development. For this reason every newborn infant is screened for congenital hypothyroidism by measuring TSH levels in blood spots (these are drops of blood, taken from a heel-prick, dried onto pieces of filter paper). A high TSH level is diagnostic of the disorder (see *Box 6.3*).

Box 6.3 Goitre

Theophrastus Bombastus von Hohenheim (1493–1541), a Swiss physician and a pioneer of medical chemistry, recognized that goitre and cretinism were related.

6.6 MEASUREMENT OF THYROID HORMONES

Total thyroid hormone levels are measured using a competitive immunoassay. Traditionally this has been performed using a radioimmunoassay (RIA), with a radioactive iodine substituted into the T_4 or T_3 molecules. Many techniques employed today use an enzyme or fluorescent label. An example is the enzyme-multiplied immunoassay technique (EMIT) which is a homogenous immunoassay technique, as outlined in *Fig. 6.3*. An EMIT assay uses a specific antibody against T_4 or T_3, depending on the assay, and T_4 or T_3 attached to an enzyme. Binding of the enzyme-labelled T_4 or T_3 to the antibody causes the active site to be blocked, thus preventing the enzyme from acting on the substrate. The enzyme reaction can be monitored spectrophotometrically. Where a low level of hormone is present in the patient's sample, the competition between the labelled hormone and patient hormone results in most of the antibody binding with labelled hormone and little patient hormone. Therefore, there will be little enzyme activity measured. Where the patient has high hormone levels, most of the antibody binding sites will capture the hormone in the sample and little labelled hormone. In this case the unbound label is active and produces a large amount of product.

Total hormone levels have to be interpreted knowing the level of binding proteins in the blood sample. This is easily achieved by adding radioactive T_3 to the sample and measuring the uptake of the isotope by the sample: the more binding protein (or available binding sites), the greater the uptake. The uptake for a given patient is expressed as a percentage of the uptake given by pooled normal serum; this is known as a T_3 uptake test (T_3U) and reflects the number of free binding sites available for thyroid hormones. From the results of the T_3 uptake test and the total T_4, the free thyroxine

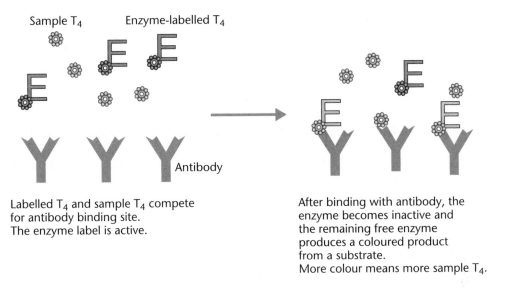

Sample T$_4$ Enzyme-labelled T$_4$

Antibody

Labelled T$_4$ and sample T$_4$ compete
for antibody binding site.
The enzyme label is active.

After binding with antibody, the
enzyme becomes inactive and
the remaining free enzyme
produces a coloured product
from a substrate.
More colour means more sample T$_4$.

Figure 6.3
The principle behind the enzyme-multiplied immunoassay technique (EMIT).

index (FTI) can be calculated, which reflects the level of the free hormone
in the sample. The calculation used is:

$$FTI = T_4 \times \%T_3U$$

Most laboratories now measure the **free hormone** levels directly, thus
avoiding the need for measuring the T$_3$ uptake. This reflects the physiological condition of the patient more accurately, as it is the free hormone that
is physiologically active. The free hormones are measured by using a labelled
analogue that competes with the free hormone in the sample for binding
sites on the antibody. This theoretically prevents dissociation of hormone
from the carrier proteins, allowing only free hormone to be measured. In
some assays this may not always have been the case.

TSH is measured with a non-competitive method using a labelled
antibody technique. Traditionally this was an immunoradiometric assay
(IRMA), using radioactive iodine as the label. Modern assays use enzyme,
fluorescent or luminescent labels. Modern assays use two monoclonal
antibodies, one specific for the α chain and the other specific for the β chain.
Using sensitive labels gives an ultrasensitive method which can measure the
extremely low levels of TSH seen in hyperthyroid patients.

Most modern clinical biochemistry laboratories measure only TSH and
free thyroxine as front-line tests. Thyroid disease can be differentiated in the
majority of patients using just these two assays.

SUGGESTED FURTHER READING

In addition to relevant chapters in the books cited in Chapters 1 and 5 the following references are recommended.

Dayan C.M. (2001) Interpretation of thyroid function tests. *The Lancet*, **357**: 619–624.
Keffer J.H. (1996) Preanalytical considerations in testing thyroid function. *Clinical Chemistry*, **42**: 125–134.
Parish N.M. and Cooke A. (2004) Mechanisms of autoimmune thyroid disease. *Drug Discovery Today: Disease Mechanisms*, **1**: 337–344.

SELF-ASSESSMENT QUESTIONS

1. Which plasma proteins are involved in transporting thyroid hormones?
2. Which two hormones control the release of thyroid hormones?
3. Which are the physiologically active hormones?
4. Which thyroid hormone is active at the cellular level?
5. What thyroid condition is characterized by high thyroxine and low TSH levels?
6. In primary hypothyroidism what would you expect the TSH level to be?
7. What is the usual cause of secondary hyperthyroidism?
8. Give an example of a homogeneous immunoassay for thyroxine.
9. Most modern laboratories measure which hormones in their thyroid screen?

Control of water and electrolyte metabolism

Learning objectives
After studying this chapter you should confidently be able to:

■ **Describe the distribution of water, sodium and potassium in the body.**
Body water is divided between the intracellular fluid and extracellular fluid. Potassium is the major intracellular cation and sodium is the major extracellular cation.

■ **Define and calculate osmolality.**
Osmolality is a measure of the concentration of dissolved particles in 1 kg of water. Osmolality is controlled by antidiuretic hormone and aldosterone.

■ **Explain the interaction of hormones controlling fluid balance.**
Antidiuretic hormone is also called arginine vasopressin. Antidiuretic hormone regulates the amount of water reabsorbed by the kidney. Aldosterone regulates the amount of sodium reabsorbed by the kidney. Aldosterone is regulated by the renin–angiotensin system.

■ **Catagorize the major disorders of water and electrolyte homeostasis.**
The lack of antidiuretic hormone is known as diabetes insipidus. A plasma sodium concentration greater than 145 mmol l^{-1} is hypernatraemia. A plasma sodium concentration less than 130 mmol l^{-1} is hyponatremia. Addison's disease is a loss of adrenal function resulting in insufficient aldosterone and cortisol production.

■ **Outline methods used to measure sodium, potassium and osmolality.**
Sodium and potassium can be measured by flame emission spectroscopy and by ion-selective electrodes. The plasma exclusion effect is an underestimation of electrolytes due to the presence of a high lipid or protein content in the sample. Electrochemical methods measure the activity of sodium or potassium ions, which is then related to the concentration.

Our body is composed mainly of water, with an average adult male containing approximately 40 litres. Dissolved in this water are many salts, nutrients and waste products. The regulation of water balance involves maintaining the correct amount of water in which these substances are dissolved. The water in our body is constantly being lost in urine, sweat and faeces, and via the lungs, and thus, in order to maintain the correct amount of water in the body, we need to drink. If we did not replace lost water we would very quickly become dehydrated, with extreme dehydration being life-threatening. The body carefully matches the loss of water with water intake by inducing the feeling of thirst. In this chapter we shall study the mechanisms that control water balance and the conditions associated with a break-down of control.

7.1 WATER BALANCE

In the body, water can be divided between two compartments: the intracellular compartment containing **intracellular fluid** (ICF) and the extracellular compartment containing **extracellular fluid** (ECF). The ECF can be further divided into interstitial fluid found between the cells and the plasma found in the circulatory system. Separating the ECF and ICF compartments is a semi-permeable cell membrane across which water can pass. Generally, solutes dissolved in the water cannot pass across the cell membrane unless there is a specific transport mechanism; for example, the entry of calcium ions into a cell is very carefully regulated. *Figure 7.1* shows the distribution of water in the body and the major electrolytes in each compartment.

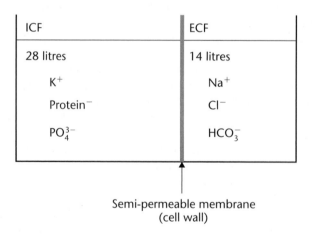

ICF	ECF
28 litres	14 litres
K^+	Na^+
$Protein^-$	Cl^-
PO_4^{3-}	HCO_3^-

Semi-permeable membrane
(cell wall)

Figure 7.1
The distribution of body water and the major solutes in the intracellular fluid and extracellular fluid compartments.

Dissolved in the water are salts, or **electrolytes**, which have an important role to play in many of the body's metabolic processes and also in the control of water balance. Electrolytes are composed of anions and cations, depending on their charge. Cations, with a positive charge, migrate towards a cathode in an electrical field and the negatively charged anions migrate towards an anode. The major electrolytes are Na^+, K^+, Ca^{2+}, Mg^{2+}, Cl^-, HCO_3^-, HPO_4^{3-} and SO_4^{2-}. These ions play an important part in the control of water balance by maintaining osmotic pressure within the fluid compartments. Other important functions of electrolytes include their role in:

- Maintenance of body pH;
- Correct functioning of muscles;
- Correct functioning of nerves;
- Acting as cofactors for enzyme reactions;
- Oxidation–reduction reactions.

The major cation in ICF is potassium and the major anion is phosphate, whereas for ECF the major cation is sodium and the major anion is chloride.

The number of dissolved particles in the body's water is measured by the **osmolality**. These particles can exist as either individual molecules, for example glucose and protein molecules, or as ions from electrolytes, for example sodium ions and chloride ions. Molecules such as glucose and proteins constitute a single particle, whereas salts such as sodium chloride dissociate to form two particles: one sodium ion and one chloride ion. The dissolved particles exert an **osmotic pressure** across the semi-permeable cell membrane, and this causes water to flow into a compartment with a higher concentration of dissolved solute relative to the other compartment. In the body, the osmotic pressure exerted by the dissolved particles will be the same on both sides of the cell membrane, which means that ICF and ECF must have the same osmolality. Any disturbance in the osmolality in one of the compartments is automatically compensated for by movement of water across the cell membrane in order to equalize the osmolality on each side of the cell membrane.

Osmolality is a measure of the concentration of dissolved particles in the blood. The unit of measurement is the **osmole**, which is defined as: the amount of solute that when dissolved in water gives the same osmotic pressure as that expected from one mole of an ideal non-ionized solute.

Osmolality is the number of osmoles dissolved in 1 kg of water. In body fluids, osmolality is measured in milliosmoles (mOsmol), with the adult reference range being 275–295 mOsmol kg^{-1}. In blood, the major elements contributing towards the osmotic pressure and hence to the osmolality are as shown in *Table 7.1*.

From *Table 7.1*, you can see that sodium and the associated anions, chloride and bicarbonate, have the greatest contribution towards the osmolality in blood, which reflects the osmolality in the ECF. Measurement of blood electrolytes can give a good indication of osmolality, and there are a number of formulae that will give a quick estimate of the osmolality, the simplest being the sodium concentration multiplied by two, which gives a rough approximation of the osmolality. There are also slightly more complicated equations that introduce concentration terms for other components; for example:

$$\text{osmolality} \approx 2[\text{Na}] + [\text{urea}] + [\text{glucose}]$$

Equations such as this are only valid if the patient does not have grossly elevated levels of protein (**hyperproteinaemia**) or lipid (**lipaemia**) in their blood (see *Box 7.1*).

Table 7.1 Approximate percentage contribution to the plasma osmolality by blood constituents

Component in plasma	Percentage contribution towards osmolality
Electrolytes	
Sodium ions	46
Chloride ions	34
Bicarbonate	9
Other anions	5
Other cations	2
Urea	1.5
Glucose	1.5
Protein	1

Box 7.1 Calculating osmolality

A patient had the following results:

Urea	4.2	mmol l^{-1}
Sodium	138	mmol l^{-1}
Potassium	4.1	mmol l^{-1}
Glucose	5.8	mmol l^{-1}

The osmolality can be calculated from:

$$(2 \times 138) + 4.2 + 5.8 = 286 \text{ mOsmol kg}^{-1}$$

7.2 THE IMPORTANCE OF SODIUM

Sodium intake in the diet is variable, up to 300 mmol per day. This is added to the total body sodium of approximately 3700 mmol in an average man, which has to be balanced by an equivalent loss. In health, the blood sodium level is carefully controlled even when intake is extremely low or extremely high. Control is achieved by regulating how much sodium is lost through the kidneys, although small losses also occur in the faeces and sweat. If sodium concentration increases, then, to maintain osmolality, water needs to be taken in to dilute the sodium. By increasing the amount of fluid in which sodium is dissolved, the fluid volume increases. If fluid volume increases in the blood vessels, this results in increased pressure within the blood vessel, i.e. increased blood pressure. One can therefore see that the control of water balance, sodium concentration and fluid volume are all interrelated, and this is reflected in the control mechanisms described below.

7.3 CONTROL OF OSMOLALITY

Osmolality reflects how much solute is dissolved in a given volume of water, and increasing the amount of solute or decreasing the volume of water will increase the osmolality. Conversely, the osmolality falls if the amount of solute is reduced or the volume of water in which the solute is dissolved is increased. In health, there are mechanisms that control the osmolality of the blood within narrow limits by adjusting the amount of solute or water present in the blood. These mechanisms are under the control of hormones that act on the kidney. The major hormones involved in maintaining plasma osmolality, and consequently water and sodium balance, are **arginine vasopressin (AVP)**, also called antidiuretic hormone (ADH), and **aldosterone**.

Arginine vasopressin regulates how much water is lost by the kidney and aldosterone regulates how much sodium is excreted by the kidney. Additionally, the thirst centre in the hypothalamus in the brain responds to increasing osmolality by inducing a feeling of thirst and thereby increasing fluid intake. As an example, how these hormones interact to restore the fluid balance in dehydration is shown in *Fig. 7.2*.

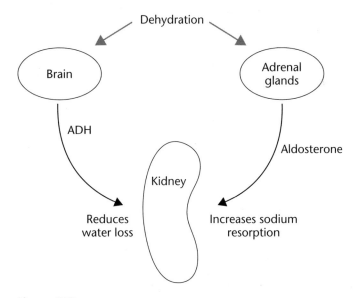

Figure 7.2
The hormone response to dehydration and the effect on the kidney to counter low fluid volume.

Arginine vasopressin

AVP is a small peptide, composed of nine amino acids, secreted by cells of the posterior pituitary gland in response to changes in osmolality. More precisely, it is the difference between the ECF and ICF osmolality that specialized cells within the hypothalamus detect, and then act to regulate AVP secretion. A falling osmolality causes a reduction in AVP secretion whereas a rising osmolality stimulates AVP release. AVP acts on the distal renal tubular cells allowing more water to be reabsorbed, producing concentrated urine with a high osmolality. In the absence of AVP, water is lost via the kidney by producing dilute urine with a low osmolality.

Aldosterone

Aldosterone is a steroid hormone synthesized and released by cells of the zona glomerulosa, in the adrenal cortex, in response to increasing blood pressure detected within the juxtaglomerular apparatus within the kidney. Release of aldosterone is under the control of the renin–angiotensin system (shown in *Fig. 7.3*), which involves kidney, lungs and the adrenal glands. In the kidney, groups of cells called the **juxtaglomerular apparatus** (JGA) are found along the afferent arterioles of the renal glomeruli. These cells of the JGA synthesize and store a proteolytic enzyme called **renin**, which is released into the blood when there is a decrease in the blood pressure within the arteriole. Renin hydrolyses a protein called angiotensinogen (synthesized in the liver), yielding **angiotensin I**. Angiotensin I is then converted to angiotensin II by the action of angiotensin-converting enzyme, found abundantly in the lung. **Angiotensin II** acts as a potent vasoconstrictor, causing an immediate increase in blood pressure. Secondly, angiotensin II stimulates cells of the zona glomerulosa to produce and secrete aldosterone, which acts to restore blood volume.

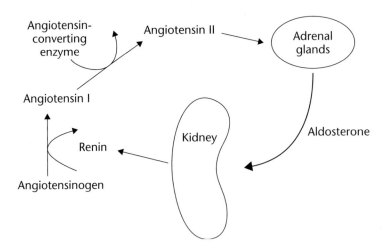

Figure 7.3
Outline of the renin–angiotensin system, which controls release of aldosterone from the adrenal gland.

Aldosterone acts on the cells of the renal tubule, causing an increase in sodium resorption. This is achieved by exchanging sodium ions in the urine for potassium or hydrogen ions, thereby increasing the sodium concentration in the blood and losing potassium and hydrogen ions in the urine. As sodium and chloride ions are generally confined to the ECF, the increase in sodium concentration due to reabsorption by the kidneys causes a rise in the ECF osmolality. This has the effect of drawing water from the ICF compartment, resulting in an increase of the ECF water content (in order to maintain osmotic neutrality between the ECF and ICF). As a consequence of the increasing fluid volume in the circulatory system, there is an increase in blood pressure. Increased blood pressure within the JGA suppresses the release of renin and therefore aldosterone levels fall.

Both aldosterone and AVP work together to maintain the plasma osmolality. At the same time, osmolality is a reflection of the fluid volume and water and electrolyte balance. Other hormones have smaller effects on water and electrolyte balance, including adrenocorticotropic hormone, cortisol and atrial natriuretic peptide.

7.4 DISORDERS OF WATER AND ELECTROLYTE BALANCE

We have seen that the most important constituents that contribute to the osmolality in blood are sodium and chloride ions. In clinical biochemistry laboratories, sodium measurements are one of the most frequently requested tests. The sodium concentration can give information about the state of hydration of the patient and may also indicate rarer conditions where there is a disorder of the hormonal control of water and electrolyte balance. Changes seen in the blood sodium concentration which are associated with water and electrolyte balance reflect the osmolality of the ECF. Abnormalities of sodium levels fall into two major categories: those characterized by high sodium concentrations and those characterized by low sodium concentrations. These are known as **hypernatraemia** and **hyponatraemia**, respectively.

Hypernatraemia (sodium >145 mmol l^{-1})

There are two circumstances which lead to hypernatraemia, and these are:

1. Dehydration resulting in increased concentration of dissolved solute particles;
2. Excess solute dissolved in the ECF.

Signs and symptoms may depend on the patient's state of hydration. Clinical signs of hypernatraemia include:

- A feeling of thirst;
- Mental confusion;
- Coma (in severe cases).

If there is water deficiency, other symptoms may include:

- Haemoconcentration resulting in raised laboratory results such as protein concentration or blood cell counts;
- Hypotension;
- Renal insufficiency.

The following discussion considers the above causes of hypernatraemia by first examining normal physiological processes and then pathological conditions. The first part considers the effects of dehydration, which can be due to a lack of fluid intake as seen in cases of severe water deprivation or in the patient who is unconscious and unable to drink. It must be appreciated that fluid is being constantly lost in sweat and via the lungs, in addition to loss in the urine. If the lost fluid is not replaced, the ECF volume drops and thus there is a lower volume of fluid in which the same amount of sodium can be dissolved. In this situation, the dehydration observed and the resulting hypernatraemia are physiological responses to the lack of fluid intake. This is the most common cause of hypernatraemia. Water is also lost if the patient has suffered from prolonged vomiting and/or diarrhoea, or has extensive burns, but in these circumstances sodium is also lost. If more water is lost relative to sodium, the result is again hypernatraemia.

Dehydration can also be caused by a pathological loss of water in the urine, as seen in the case of a patient who has a lack of AVP; this is known as **diabetes insipidus**. These patients are unable to conserve water and produce large volumes of dilute urine. This reduces the blood volume, resulting in hypernatraemia.

The second group of conditions that give rise to hypernatraemia are those where there is an increased amount of sodium dissolved in the blood. This could be induced by giving the patient too much sodium intravenously, as part of the treatment for another condition. Rarely, hypernatraemia is caused by an inappropriate overproduction of aldosterone, known as **Conn's syndrome**. An overproduction of cortisol, as seen in **Cushing's syndrome**, can also give rise to hypernatraemia (see *Box 7.2*).

Box 7.2 Cushing's syndrome

Cushing's syndrome is named after Harvey William Cushing (1869–1939), a neurosurgeon who worked on the removal of brain tumours. He also studied the pathology of the pituitary gland and showed that Cushing's syndrome could be associated with a particular type of pituitary tumour.

Hyponatraemia (sodium <130 mmol l⁻¹)

There are two circumstances that lead to hyponatraemia, and these are:

1. Overhydration, resulting in solute particles being diluted;
2. Reduced number of solute particles being present in the ECF.

Symptoms may depend on whether there is an excess of water contributing to the hyponatraemia. Clinical signs of hyponatraemia include:

- Headache;
- Confusion and fits (if severe).

If there is an excess of water, other symptoms may include:

- Oedema;
- Hypertension, which can lead to cardiac failure;
- Haemodilution resulting in low laboratory results due to the dilution effect.

In the first cause of hyponatraemia listed, there is an excess of water in the ECF. This increases the fluid volume and therefore the sodium ions in the ECF are diluted. To maintain an osmotic balance water is drawn into the ICF. Overhydration can occur as a consequence of reduced water output, as may be seen in patients with renal failure, where urine is not produced and also in the **syndrome of inappropriate antidiuretic hormone** (SIADH). In this condition, the production and release of AVP is stimulated by non-osmotic factors such as pain, hypoglycaemia or hypotension. AVP acts on the kidneys causing water retention and consequently, by dilution, hyponatraemia. This is commonly seen in conditions such as cancer, infections or major trauma.

To maintain an efficient excretion of water via the kidneys, there needs to be sufficient blood pressure to filter blood in the kidney to form urine. Blood pressure is related to blood volume, and a reduction in volume reduces the blood pressure. Another factor is protein in the blood, which helps to retain blood volume by maintaining the oncotic pressure within the blood vessels. Where there is insufficient protein the blood volume drops. In conditions where the blood pressure or blood volume is reduced, for example in cardiac failure or nephrotic syndrome (where a large amount of protein is lost in the urine), a reduced volume of urine is formed and water is retained. In these conditions, sodium is also retained due to stimulation of aldosterone release and its effects on the kidney. When retention of water is relatively greater than that of sodium, hyponatraemia results. If fluid accumulates in the interstitial compartment, it causes swelling of the tissues, which is known as **oedema**.

Water overload can also be caused by an increased water intake. This is sometimes seen in a patient who is a compulsive water drinker, or after inappropriate intravenous therapy.

Hyponatraemia can also be caused by a lowered amount of sodium in the body. This could be due to excessive loss or insufficient intake. The loss of sodium ions, which leads to sodium depletion, is usually due to a pathological process. Sodium is predominantly lost in the urine or via the gastrointestinal tract. Pathological urinary losses occur when the patient has a deficiency of the hormone aldosterone, which is generally a result of adrenal failure; this is called **Addison's disease** (cortisol is also deficient). Without sufficient aldosterone, sodium ions are not reabsorbed in the kidney and initially water is also lost with the sodium, thereby depleting the

---

Box 7.3 Addison's disease

Addison's disease is named after Thomas Addison (1793–1860) who was one of the founders of endocrinology. He linked Addison's disease with changes in the suprarenal capsules, now called the adrenal glands.

ECF. As the blood volume falls, release of AVP is stimulated, which causes water retention and results in worsening hyponatraemia. Gastrointestinal losses occur if the patient suffers from severe vomiting or diarrhoea. Insufficient intake of sodium leading to hyponatraemia is only seen in rare cases (see *Box 7.3*).

Table 7.2 gives a summary of the changes seen in some of the conditions leading to hyponatraemia and hypernatraemia.

Table 7.2 Summary of changes seen in some of the conditions leading to hyponatraemia and hypernatraemia*

	AVP	Aldosterone	Plasma Na	Water loss in urine
Dehydration	↑	↑	↑	↓
Overhydration	↓	↓	↓	↑
Diabetes insipidus	↑	↑	↑	↑
Conn's syndrome	↑	↑	↑	↓
SIADH	↑	↓/N	↓	↓
Addison's disease	↑	↓	↓	↓/N

*Bold arrows represent pathological changes due to loss of regulation of the hormone.

7.5 POTASSIUM

Potassium is measured in the clinical biochemistry laboratory in the same group of tests as sodium, forming part of the **electrolyte profile**. It is an important measurement as large changes in the blood potassium concentration can be life-threatening. As we have discussed previously in this chapter, potassium is the most important intracellular cation, with approximately 3500 mmol in the ICF and 55 mmol in the ECF (see *Box 7.4*).

Intake of potassium is highly varied but the blood concentration of sodium is kept within reasonably tight limits of 3.6–5.0 mmol l^{-1}. The blood concentration is maintained principally by the kidney. In health, excess potassium is excreted in the urine; the potassium ions in the kidney tubule cells are exchanged for sodium ions from the glomerular filtrate. Hydrogen ions are also exchanged for sodium ions, which means that the relative

> **Box 7.4 Sodium and potassium**
>
> Sodium (atomic number 11, atomic weight 23, boiling point 883°C) is the seventh most abundant element in the earth's crust. Potassium (atomic number 19, atomic weight 39, boiling point 762°C) is also a common constituent of the earth's crust. Both these reactive alkali metals were first isolated by Sir Humphry Davy in 1807.

amounts of hydrogen and potassium in the tubule cells influence the amount of potassium excreted. This exchange of sodium for potassium is stimulated by the hormone aldosterone. Thus, there are three factors that can influence the amount of potassium lost through the kidney:

- The amount of sodium in the glomerular filtrate available for exchange;
- The hydrogen ion concentration;
- The aldosterone level.

Small amounts of potassium are lost in the faeces, but this may increase significantly in pathological conditions where there is increased, abnormal gastrointestinal loss.

Potassium levels are also greatly influenced by the acid–base balance of the patient (see Chapter 14). If an excess of hydrogen ions accumulates within a cell, to maintain neutrality of charge across the membrane potassium ions move from the cell into the ECF, causing the blood concentration of potassium to rise. Conversely, potassium ions move from the ECF into cells when there is a reduction in the hydrogen ion concentration within the cell.

7.6 DISORDERS OF POTASSIUM METABOLISM

As with sodium, we will consider those conditions that lead to an excess and a deficiency of potassium in the blood. The presence of a high concentration of potassium in the blood is called **hyperkalaemia** and a low concentration is called **hypokalaemia**.

Hyperkalaemia

Hyperkalaemia is defined as a blood concentration of potassium greater than 5.0 mmol l^{-1}. Concentrations greater than 7.0 mmol l^{-1} are life-threatening as they can lead to a cardiac arrest. Symptoms of hyperkalaemia include:

- Muscle weakness;
- Paraesthesia;
- Abnormal ECG;
- Cardiac arrest.

A high potassium concentration in the blood can be due to either an increase of potassium ions entering the ECF or an inefficient secretion of excess potassium ions. Since potassium is the major intercellular cation, cellular damage can release large amounts of potassium into the ECF. For example, trauma and cancer, where there is cell destruction, often give rise to hyperkalaemia. Blood samples that are haemolysed give a high potassium concentration in the plasma sample; this is an artefactual result because potassium has been released into the sample from the red blood cells. A similar artefactual high potassium result is seen where blood samples have been left overnight before separating the serum or plasma from the blood cells. Another situation where the release of potassium from cells into the ECF occurs is in those patients who have an excess of hydrogen ions (known as **acidosis** – see Chapter 14). In acidosis, potassium from within cells is redistributed to the ECF, thereby raising the blood potassium concentration. Finally, an increase in potassium concentration could be seen during poorly controlled intravenous therapy where potassium is being given to the patient.

Hyperkalaemia resulting from inefficient excretion of potassium is seen in renal disease where an insufficient volume of urine is being formed; this is associated with a low glomerular filtration rate (see Chapter 17). As we have discussed, potassium is exchanged for sodium in the distal renal tubule, under the control of aldosterone. Hypoaldosteronism (as seen in **Addison's disease**) results in an inefficient exchange of ions, leading to potassium retention and the loss of sodium ions.

Hypokalaemia

Hypokalaemia is a blood potassium concentration less than 3.6 mmol l^{-1} and usually occurs as a result of excessive loss of potassium from the body. Symptoms include:

- Muscle weakness;
- Cardiac arrhythmias;
- Abnormal ECG.

Loss of potassium can be due to gastrointestinal losses such as prolonged vomiting and/or diarrhoea, or renal losses. Renal losses of potassium are excessive where the patient has high levels of sodium in the glomerular filtrate or has hyperaldosteronism, for example Conn's syndrome, causing excessive sodium–potassium exchange. Certain drugs such as thiazide diuretics promote sodium–potassium exchange in the distal tubule, thereby increasing potassium loss in the urine. Potassium can be lost from the ECF into the ICF leading to hypokalaemia although there is no overall loss of body potassium. This redistribution of potassium occurs in those patients with a depletion of hydrogen ions, i.e. **alkalosis** (see Chapter 14), where potassium ions enter the cell to maintain electroneutrality. In situations where there is an inadequate intake of potassium, hypokalaemia can develop, as in cases of prolonged starvation.

7.7 MEASUREMENT OF SODIUM AND POTASSIUM

Sodium and potassium measurements are probably the most commonly requested tests, along with their associated analytes, in the clinical biochemistry laboratory. They are part of the urea and electrolyte groups of tests, known as Us and Es. There are two main techniques used to measure these ions: the first is by flame emission spectroscopy and the second is an electrochemical technique using an ion-selective electrode.

Electrolyte exclusion effect

Electrolytes are dissolved in the water fraction of plasma – plasma water. Proteins and lipids make up the solid fraction of plasma, which is usually about 8% of the plasma volume. Thus, 92% of plasma is plasma water, which contains the dissolved electrolytes. When a sample is analysed, in the volume taken, for example 100 μl, the amount of electrolyte measured is contained in the 92 μl of plasma water. If the patient has very high levels of protein or lipid, the fraction of plasma water in a given volume of sample will be lower and therefore there will be less electrolyte available for measurement. In this situation, an artificially low concentration of electrolyte is recorded, despite a normal concentration of electrolyte in the plasma water; this is known as the **electrolyte exclusion effect**. All methods that measure the concentration of electrolyte in a given volume of sample are subject to this effect, and this includes flame emission spectroscopy and indirect measurement using ion-selective electrodes (discussed below). *Figure 7.4* shows the electrolyte exclusion effect.

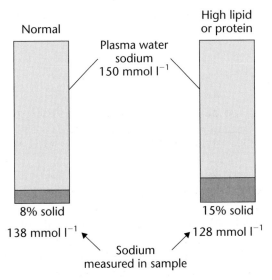

Figure 7.4
The principle involved in pseudohyponatraemia.

Pseudohyponatraemia occurs when a low sodium concentration is measured in a patient with very high levels of protein or lipid present in the plasma, despite having a normal concentration of sodium in the plasma water. If the osmolality were to be measured in these patients, it would be normal.

Flame emission spectroscopy

Often called flame photometry, this once-routine technique is now used as a back-up or for urinary analysis. In this technique, the sample is introduced into a flame, which excites the outer electrons of the sodium and potassium atoms. Electrons gain energy from the flame, pushing them to a higher, unstable energy level. As the excited electrons lose energy, falling back to their original ground state, a photon of light is emitted at a characteristic wavelength. The greater the concentration of sodium or potassium in the sample, the greater the number of electrons that are excited and decay to give photons of light. The concentration is proportional to the intensity of light emitted at the characteristic wavelength of that metal. The light is usually measured using a photocell. This technique is similar to the simple flame test for metals, each metal showing a characteristic colour of flame. Because each metal emits light at a characteristic wavelength, both sodium and potassium can be measured simultaneously. *Table 7.3* shows the colour of the flame observed and the wavelength of the major emission band which is used to measure the metal concentration for sodium, potassium and some other metals measured by flame emission.

Table 7.3 Flame colour and wavelength of the major emission band for metals measured by flame emission spectroscopy

Metal	Flame colour	Wavelength (nm)
Sodium	Yellow	589
Potassium	Lilac	768
Lithium	Red	671
Barium	Apple green	553
Caesium	Red	852

Ion-selective electrodes

Modern clinical analysers used to process the majority of samples arriving in the clinical biochemistry laboratory use an ion-selective electrode (ISE) to measure the concentration of sodium and potassium. When using electrochemical methods, it is more accurate to refer to the **activity** of the sodium or potassium ions rather than concentration. Activity is then related to the concentration in the sample.

An ISE consists of a membrane with the sample on one side and a reference solution on the other. In the presence of specific ions in the sample a potential is generated across the membrane, due to an uneven distribution of charge on either side of the membrane. The potential is measured against a reference electrode built into the ion-selective electrode. The most commonly used ISE is the pH electrode, which measures hydrogen ion activity across a glass membrane. The potential generated in millivolts is converted into pH units for the read-out scale on the pH meter. By changing this glass membrane, the pH electrode can be made selective for other ions, for example sodium. The membrane can be made from special formulations of glass, or can be made from single crystals or from thin-film plastic membranes (e.g. PVC) containing a specific charge carrier.

ISEs can be used in two ways, namely the indirect method and the direct method. In the indirect method, the sample is diluted in a high ionic strength buffer before the measurement is made. In contrast, direct methods use undiluted sample at the electrode surface. Due to the large dilution of a fixed sample volume in high ionic strength buffers, indirect methods in effect measure concentration directly and suffer from the electrolyte exclusion effect. In contrast, direct methods measure the activity of electrolytes in the plasma water of an undiluted sample and therefore are independent of sample volume and are unaffected by the electrolyte exclusion effect.

Sodium electrodes

Altering the composition of the glass membrane by preparing the glass from silicon, sodium and aluminium oxides in the ratio of 71:11:18 causes the electrode to become selective for sodium ions. This does not mean that the electrode is specific, but rather that it reacts most strongly to sodium ions.

Potassium electrodes

Potassium-selective electrodes incorporate valinomycin into the membrane of the ISE. Valinomycin binds potassium ions, making an ISE highly selective for potassium.

SUGGESTED FURTHER READING

In addition to relevant chapters in the text books cited in Chapters 1 and 5 the following references are recommended.

Atherton J.C. (2006) Regulation of fluid and electrolyte balance by the kidney. *Anaesthesia & Intensive Care Medicine*, **7**: 227–233.
Brewster U.C. and Perazella M.A. (2004) The renin-angiotensin-aldosterone system and the kidney: effects on kidney disease. *American Journal of Medicine*, **116**: 263–272.

Campbell I. (2006) Physiology of fluid balance. *Anaesthesia & Intensive Care Medicine*, **7**: 462–465.

Weiss M., Dullenkopf A. and Moehrlen U. (2004) Evaluation of an improved blood-conserving POCT sampling system. *Clinical Biochemistry*, **37**: 977–984.

SELF-ASSESSMENT QUESTIONS

1. What is the unit of measurement for the concentration of dissolved particles in blood?
2. Which is the most important organ controlling sodium concentration in the blood?
3. Which are the two most important hormones involved in water and sodium balance?
4. What is the effect of aldosterone on cells of the renal tubule?
5. How is aldosterone release regulated?
6. Patients who lack antidiuretic hormone have which disease?
7. Which hormones are lacking in Addison's disease?
8. Why are haemolysed blood samples not suitable for plasma potassium analysis?
9. Which two different methods can be used to measure sodium and potassium?
10. Do direct methods of measurement using an ion-selective electrode suffer from the electrolyte exclusion effect?

Control of calcium metabolism

Learning objectives
After studying this chapter you should confidently be able to:

■ **Describe where calcium is found in the body.**
Calcium is widely distributed in the body, mainly in the bones, and is in a state of flux between bone and body fluids. It is free 'ionized' calcium that is physiologically active. Calcium is important in cell signalling.

■ **Outline the actions of the main hormones involved in controlling calcium homeostasis.**
Calcium levels are controlled by parathyroid hormone and 1,25-DHCC, acting on kidneys, bones and the small intestine. Parathyroid hormone acts on the kidney and bone to raise the plasma calcium concentration. 1,25-DHCC acts on the small intestine and bone to raise the plasma calcium concentration.

■ **Categorize the major types of disease which disturb calcium homeostasis.**
Disorders of calcium metabolism can lead to hypercalcaemia or hypocalcaemia. Hypercalcaemia (calcium concentration >2.8 mmol l^{-1}) is found in malignancy and in primary and tertiary hyperparathyroidism. Hypocalcaemia (calcium concentration <2.1 mmol l^{-1}) is found in hypoparathyroidism, vitamin D deficiency and renal disease.

■ **Describe the methods used to measure plasma calcium.**
Calcium can be measured using atomic absorption, dye-binding methods and ion-selective electrodes.

In this chapter we shall see how the concentration of calcium in the blood is controlled by the interaction of parathyroid hormone and cholecalciferol, a metabolite of vitamin D. Unlike the hormones discussed in the previous chapters, there is no hormonal axis as these hormones act directly on various organs to maintain the blood calcium concentration within tight limits.

8.1 CALCIUM

Calcium, derived mainly from dairy products, is the fifth most common element and the major divalent cation in the body, with the vast majority found in bone. There is approximately 1 kg (about 25 mol) of calcium in an adult of which 99% is found in bones and teeth as crystalline hydroxy-apatite, whilst the blood contains approximately 800 mg (20 mmol) of calcium. This calcium is not static but is in a continual state of flux with calcium being absorbed through the gut, moving in and out of the bone, and being lost in the urine via the kidneys. Approximately 10% of bone is 'turned over' every year.

Calcium in the blood is found almost exclusively in the plasma where it exists in three forms:

- 45% protein bound;
- 10% complexed with citrate, phosphate, lactate and bicarbonate;
- 45% ionized or 'free'.

It is the free, unbound fraction which is physiologically active and is important for:

- Maintaining skeletal tissue;
- Muscle contraction;
- Controlling cell functions;
- Release of neurotransmitters;
- Blood coagulation;
- Cell adhesion.

As calcium is so important in the control of many intracellular and extra-cellular signalling pathways, the concentration necessary to maintain health is closely regulated (see *Box 8.1*).

Box 8.1 Calcium and magnesium

The physiologically important divalent cations are calcium and magnesium. Calcium was first isolated in 1808 by Sir Humphry Davy. It is a reactive metal with relative atomic mass 40.08 and atomic number 20. Magnesium was also first isolated by Sir Humphry Davy in the same year. Its relative atomic mass is 24.3 and its atomic number is 12.

8.2 CALCIUM CONTROL

Plasma calcium levels are maintained within fine limits by the action of two hormones. The most important of these is **parathyroid hormone** (PTH) and the second is **1,25-dihydroxycholecalciferol** (1,25-DHCC). *Figure 8.1* shows the inter-relationships between these hormones and the organs they act upon to maintain the blood calcium level between 2.25 and 2.88 mmol l^{-1}.

Parathyroid hormone

PTH is a single-chain polypeptide made of 84 amino acids (molecular weight 9.5 kDa) produced by the **parathyroid glands**. It is formed from pre-

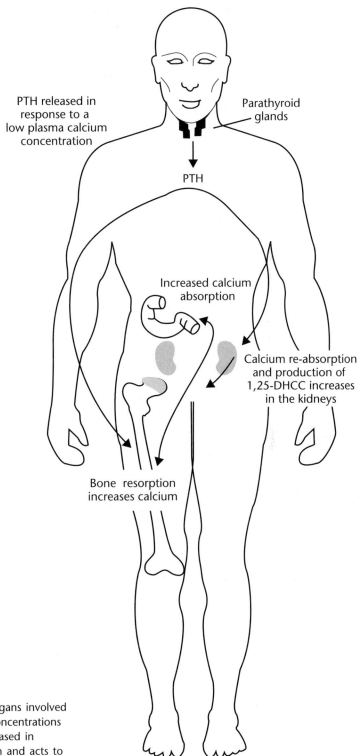

PTH released in
response to a
low plasma calcium
concentration

Parathyroid
glands

PTH

Increased calcium
absorption

Calcium re-absorption
and production of
1,25-DHCC increases
in the kidneys

Bone resorption
increases calcium

Figure 8.1
The relationship between the organs involved
in maintaining blood calcium concentrations
within narrow limits. PTH is released in
response to a low blood calcium and acts to
raise the calcium concentration.

proPTH (115 amino acids) which is converted to pro-PTH (90 amino acids) and then to PTH. The biological activity of PTH is found in the first 34 N-terminal amino acids and the biological half-life of the protein is approximately 15–30 minutes.

There are four parathyroid glands situated in the neck close to the thyroid. The 'chief' cells are responsible for the storage and secretion of PTH. Secretion of PTH is stimulated in response to a low free-calcium concentration in the blood. PTH acts to increase calcium levels in the blood by:

■ Stimulating osteoclasts in the bone to release calcium from bone stores into the extracellular fluid. Phosphate and hydroxyproline levels also rise, as these are released from the bone at the same time;
■ Increasing absorption of calcium in the kidney. Phosphate reabsorption is decreased, leading to the lowering of plasma levels due to phosphate being lost in the urine – phosphaturia;
■ Increasing synthesis of 1,25-DHCC.

The result of PTH action is an increase in free and total plasma calcium with a decrease in plasma phosphate levels. As circulating levels of **free calcium** increase, a negative feedback system reduces the amount of PTH released by the parathyroid gland.

A second form of PTH called **parathyroid hormone-related peptide (PTHrp)** has been identified. This protein has the same first 13 N-terminal amino acids as PTH, but is a larger protein, containing between 139 and 173 amino acids. PTHrp has been shown to be synthesized by many tumours that lead to hypercalcaemia, although the protein has a number of important physiological roles in health (see *Box 8.2*).

Box 8.2 Reference ranges

The reference range for PTH is 29–85 pmol l^{-1}. It is usually measured using an immunoassay.
The reference range for 1,25-DHCC is 40.9–141.8 pmol l^{-1}, and it is measured using a protein binding assay employing vitamin D binding receptors extracted from homogenized chick intestinal mucosa, bovine thymus or rat osteosarcoma.

1,25-Dihydroxycholecalciferol

1,25-DHCC is a metabolite of **vitamin D_3** (cholecalciferol) which is taken in the diet or formed in the skin by the action of sunlight on 7-dehydro-cholesterol. *Figure 8.2* shows a simplified diagram of the metabolic pathways and the factors controlling the synthesis of 1,25-DHCC.

The liver synthesizes 25-hydroxycholecalciferol (25-HCC) which is released into the circulation. In the kidney 25-HCC is further hydroxylated to 1,25-DHCC which is biologically active, or 24,25-DHCC which is inactive. High levels of PTH and low levels of calcium and phosphate activate the synthesis of 1,25-DHCC, which is highly potent in its actions, resulting in:

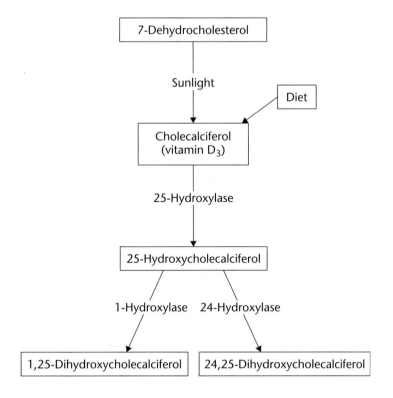

Figure 8.2
The formation of 1,25-dihydroxycholecalciferol.

- Increased calcium and phosphate uptake in the intestine;
- Increased calcium resorption from bone, acting synergistically with PTH;
- Increased absorption of calcium by the kidneys.

The result of 1,25-DHCC production is an increase in plasma concentrations of total and free calcium. The combined action of PTH and 1,25-DHCC increases levels of calcium in the blood which in turn raises the levels of calcium excreted in the urine and this is despite increased calcium uptake by the kidneys.

Calcitonin

This hormone has a minor role in the control of calcium metabolism and may be more important in the foetus and young child. It is produced by the C cells in the thyroid and is a 32 amino acid polypeptide. Elevated free-calcium levels stimulate the release of calcitonin whereas low calcium levels are inhibitory. The effect of this hormone is to inhibit the release of calcium from bone.

8.3   PHOSPHATE

Phosphate is an important anion found throughout the body both intra-
and extracellularly. Intracellular phosphate is associated with organic
molecules such as phospholipids and energy-producing compounds such as
ATP. Phosphate is also important in cell-signalling pathways and in the
regulation of some metabolic pathways. Extracellular phosphate is primarily inorganic in the form of hydrogen and dihydrogen phosphates. Here they
have a role of acting as buffers. Blood levels show a diurnal rhythm and are
influenced by meals, so the reference ranges are based on fasting blood
samples. The reference range for an adult is 0.8–1.4 mmol l^{-1}. This range is
age-related. Measurement of phosphate is useful in the investigation of
hyper- and hypocalcaemia as it can aid in differential diagnosis.

8.4   DISORDERS OF CALCIUM METABOLISM

Assuming a good supply of calcium and vitamin D, normal calcium
homeostasis is maintained by the **parathyroid gland**, the **kidneys**, the **intestine** and the **bone** as seen in *Fig. 8.3*. Disease or abnormal functioning of
any of the four organs associated with control, input, output or storage of
calcium will give rise to abnormal calcium concentrations in the blood. This
in turn will affect the function calcium has in the body, resulting in the

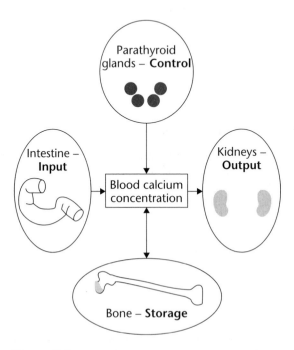

Figure 8.3
The role of organs involved in the control of calcium concentration.

Box 8.3 Calcium disorder tests

In a routine clinical biochemistry laboratory a typical test profile for the investigation of a suspected calcium disorder, perhaps related to bone or kidney disease, would include the following:

- Calcium;
- Phosphate;
- Alkaline phosphatase;
- Total protein;
- Albumin.

---

symptoms observed in the patient. There are two main categories of disease which are reflected in pathological changes in the calcium concentration in the blood: those conditions which result in high levels of calcium – **hypercalcaemia**; and those which result in low levels of calcium in the blood – **hypocalcaemia** (see *Box 8.3*).

Before we discuss these, recall that approximately 50% of calcium in the blood is bound to protein, with the most important protein being **albumin**. If for any reason the albumin concentration is abnormal, the total calcium concentration will be altered to reflect this, even though the unbound, free calcium is still normal. For example, if the albumin is low (as might be the case in many hospitalized patients), the measured total calcium concentration will also be low, despite having a normal free-calcium concentration. Conversely, a high albumin level (due to dehydration or stasis during blood collection) will increase the observed total calcium concentration because the protein-bound fraction is raised; again the free calcium is normal. This has important implications in the interpretation of total calcium results, as the albumin concentration needs to be considered. Many hospitals apply a correction factor to their total calcium results, producing a **corrected calcium**. This correction has the effect of normalizing the albumin to 47 g l^{-1} and adjusting the calcium concentration to reflect this. The equation for this is:

Corrected calcium (mmol l^{-1}) = total calcium + 0.02(47 – albumin in g l^{-1})

This equation increases or decreases the calcium concentration by 0.1 mmol l^{-1} for every 5 g l^{-1} the albumin is below or above 47 g l^{-1}, respectively (see *Box 8.4*).

Box 8.4 Corrected calcium concentration

A patient has a total calcium level of 2.36 mmol l^{-1} and an albumin concentration of 37 g l^{-1}. The corrected calcium is given by:

Total calcium + 0.02(47 – albumin in g l^{-1})
2.36 + 0.02(47 – 37)
2.36 + 0.02 × 10 = 2.36 + 0.2 = 2.56

The corrected calcium is therefore 2.56; the formula has elevated the measured calcium value from the low end towards the middle of the reference range, due to the 'lowish' albumin concentration.

Another factor influencing the calcium status of a patient is the **acid–base** balance (see Chapter 14). The binding of calcium to protein is pH dependent, and acidosis causes increased levels of free calcium due to the dissociation of calcium from protein at low pH. Conversely, in alkalosis, reduced levels of free calcium are found, as more calcium is protein-bound. It is the free, unbound fraction that is physiologically active so in acid–base disturbances, symptoms of hypo- or hypercalcaemia are seen, despite having a normal total calcium concentration.

Hypercalcaemia

Hypercalcaemia is defined as a corrected plasma calcium concentration greater than 2.8 mmol l^{-1}. A level greater than 3.5 mmol l^{-1} is life-threatening and immediate action is required. The symptoms of hypercalcaemia include:

■ Lethargy, confusion and depression;
■ Abdominal pain, nausea and vomiting;
■ Renal problems such as renal stones;
■ Thirst and polyuria;
■ Cardiac arrhythmias.

If the condition is long-standing it will result in demineralization of the bones and in some patients the formation of renal stones. Conditions resulting in hypercalcaemia are classified below according to the organ where the main defect in calcium homeostasis occurs.

Parathyroid gland

A PTH-secreting adenoma in the parathyroid gland is a common cause of hypercalcaemia. This is a benign tumour, which synthesizes and secretes PTH with no feedback control – the autonomous secretion of PTH. This is primary hyperparathyroidism. The PTH has the normal physiological effects on its target tissues, resulting in high blood calcium concentrations. In normal patients with a high calcium level the PTH would be suppressed to undetectable amounts, but patients with primary hyperparathyroidism have inappropriately raised levels of PTH. The parathyroid may also secrete PTH without negative feedback control following prolonged stimulation of the parathyroid gland by low calcium levels; this is known as tertiary hyperparathyroidism.

Hyperparathyroidism also affects phosphate levels, with 50% of patients having a low phosphate concentration in the blood. However, the phosphate concentration may be normal, especially if the patient has renal impairment (which could be caused by the high calcium level).

Kidney

Long-standing renal disease can induce tertiary hypoparathyroidism (see above). Mild hypercalcaemia is also associated with thiazide diuretic therapy, which causes calcium to be retained in the blood.

Intestine

Excessive intake of calcium or vitamin D can cause hypercalcaemia. A rare situation called milk-alkali syndrome can lead to hypercalcaemia where there is an increased absorption of calcium following a large intake of calcium (in milk) with antacids containing bicarbonate.

Bone

Occasionally hypercalcaemia may be seen in patients with Paget's disease, especially if they are immobilized.

Hypercalcaemia of malignancy

This is the most common cause of increased calcium concentrations in hospitalized patients. It occurs in 10–20% of patients with malignant disease. Examples of conditions associated with hypercalcaemia include cancer of the breast, prostate, bronchus or kidney, and multiple myeloma. The hypercalcaemia is due to the action of tumour cells that can:

■ Metastasize to the bone and resorb bone directly, releasing calcium;
■ Activate osteoclasts and bone breakdown via the prostaglandins produced by some tumours;
■ Produce PTHrP, which is synthesized by the tumour cells and has the physiological actions of PTH.

Hypocalcaemia

Hypocalcaemia is defined as a corrected plasma calcium concentration of less than 2.1 mmol l^{-1}. Symptoms of hypocalcaemia include:

■ Tetany due to increased neuromuscular activity;
■ Cataracts;
■ Psychiatric symptoms such as depression.

Again, diseases associated with hypocalcaemia can be classified according to the organ where the main defect in calcium homeostasis occurs.

Parathyroid gland

Destruction of the parathyroid gland due to an autoimmune disease, infection, infiltration by a tumour or damage following surgery to the neck will result in an inability to manufacture PTH, resulting in hypoparathyroidism. Here the free-calcium concentration is low but insufficient PTH is synthesized in response to this stimulus. The PTH level is inappropriately low for the low calcium concentration. A low magnesium concentration (<0.4 mmol l^{-1}) can also give the same picture, but this would be rare.

Kidney

Kidney disease results in the loss of 1,25-DHCC synthesis, resulting in a diminished ability to raise calcium levels in response to hypocalcaemia. Also, PTH may not be effective, resulting in loss of calcium in the urine and retention of phosphate. Low calcium due to kidney disease stimulates the parathyroid to produce high levels of PTH to restore calcium levels (secondary hyperparathyroidism) with limited success. Chronic renal failure may lead to tertiary hyperparathyroidism and raised calcium levels from bone desorption. The lack of 1,25-DHCC also reduces the absorption of calcium in the gut.

Intestine

Hypocalcaemia can develop in cases of malabsorption or if there is a deficiency of calcium or vitamin D in the diet and little exposure to sunlight. Prolonged deficiencies will lead to rickets in children and osteomalacia in adults. With vitamin D deficiency there is no production of 1,25-DHCC and, subsequently, PTH is released (secondary hyperparathyroidism) in an effort to raise calcium levels in the blood. PTH acts on the kidney causing reabsorption of calcium and loss of phosphate into the urine (cf. phosphate levels in renal disease; see above). Long-standing liver disease also inhibits absorption of vitamin D, the effects of which may be exacerbated by a reduced ability to produce 25-HCC.

Pseudohypoparathyroidism

This is a rare condition where there is a defect in the PTH receptors on the surfaces of bone and kidney cells. The cells do not recognize PTH and thus it has no action. This results in falling calcium levels which in turn stimulate the parathyroid gland to produce more PTH. Therefore these patients have low calcium, high phosphate and high PTH levels.

Table 8.1 gives a summary of the major changes that may be observed in some of the conditions leading to hyper- and hypocalcaemia.

Table 8.1 Changes seen in blood measurements of PTH, phosphate and 1,25-DHCC for diseases associated with hypercalcaemia and hypocalcaemia

	PTH	Phosphate	1,25-DHCC
Hypercalcaemia			
Primary hyperparathyroidism	↑	↓	↑
Tertiary hyperparathyroidism	↑	↑	↓
(chronic renal failure)			
Malignancy	↓	↓	
Vitamin D toxicity	↓	N	N
Hypocalcaemia			
Hypoparathyroidism	↓	↑	↓
Pseudohyperparathyroidism	↑	↑	↓
Secondary hyperparathyroidism			
Vitamin D deficiency and malabsorption	↑	↓	↓
Renal failure	↑	↑	↓

N, normal levels.

8.5   MEASUREMENT OF CALCIUM

There have been many different methods described for measuring calcium in the routine laboratory. These can be divided into:

■ Atomic absorption spectrophotometry;
■ Dye-binding techniques;
■ Electrochemical methods.

Atomic absorption spectrophotometry

Atomic absorption spectrophotometry (AAS) is a technique where the sample forms free calcium atoms when introduced into a flame or furnace. Monochromatic light is passed through the cloud of calcium atoms that absorb energy from the light. The monochromatic light produced by a hollow cathode lamp, has to be of a particular wavelength (422.7 nm) in order for the calcium atoms to absorb the light. The amount of light absorbed depends on the concentration of calcium in the sample: high calcium concentrations absorb more light and therefore give higher readings. By using different hollow cathode lamps, each producing its own characteristic monochromatic light, different metals can be measured in a sample. *Table 8.2* gives the wavelengths of light used to measure some other metals by AAS in a clinical biochemistry laboratory. *Figure 8.4* shows a diagram of an atomic absorption spectrophotometer.

Table 8.2 Wavelengths of light emitted by hollow cathode lamps used in atomic absorption spectroscopy to measure some of the clinically important metals

Metal	Wavelength emitted by hollow cathode lamp (nm)
Calcium	422.7
Copper	324.8
Lead	217.0 or 283.3
Magnesium	285.2
Zinc	213.9

AAS is a quick and sensitive technique but requires expensive atomic absorption instrumentation. A further disadvantage is the relatively low throughput, making it an unsuitable technique in a modern diagnostic laboratory. However, it is often found in larger laboratories performing urine analysis and research laboratories requiring a sensitive technique.

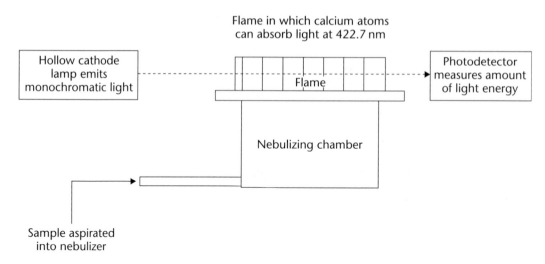

Flame in which calcium atoms can absorb light at 422.7 nm

| Hollow cathode lamp emits monochromatic light | Flame | Photodetector measures amount of light energy |

Nebulizing chamber

Sample aspirated into nebulizer

Figure 8.4
The principle of atomic absorption spectroscopy.

Dye-binding techniques

There are a number of metal-complexing dyes that change colour on binding to calcium. These are often pH dependent and may suffer from interference from other divalent cations, although this problem can be minimized by additives. The advantage of these techniques is that they can be easily automated and rely on simple absorption spectrophotometry, which measures the intensity of the colour formed. An example of a metal-binding dye used to measure calcium in plasma samples is *o*-cresolphthalein, which produces a coloured chromophore that can be measured at 578 nm. Newer techniques involving dry chemistry react the sample with Arsenazo III and the coloured product is measured by reflectance spectrophotometry at 680 nm.

Electrochemical methods

These methods use an ion-specific electrode (ISE) to measure the activity of ionized calcium, which is translated into a concentration. The advantage of using an ISE is that the physiologically active calcium is being measured, which should reflect the clinical picture more accurately without having to worry about the protein concentration. A dedicated instrument for measuring ionized calcium is required, although some large multichannel analysers use an ISE to measure the ionized calcium. The disadvantages of calcium-selective electrodes are that they suffer from interference from other divalent cations such as magnesium, they are pH dependent and they can suffer from other chemical interference such as surfactants, ethanol and chelating agents. Because the free-calcium concentration is dependent on the blood pH, special collection techniques are required so that the blood pH does not change. This requires anaerobic collection or the pH to be adjusted to the patient's pH at the time of collection – this is a complicated and time-consuming task.

Despite the potential advantage of measuring the physiological active component, ISE measurement of calcium has not been widely implemented. This is probably due to the complicated procedure used for collecting the samples and the fact that many laboratories are now employing instrumentation that uses dry chemistry.

SUGGESTED FURTHER READING

In addition to relevant chapters in the text books cited in Chapters 1 and 5 the following references are recommended.

Barth J.H., Fiddy J.B. and Payne R.B. (1996) Adjustment of serum total calcium for albumin concentration: effects of non-linearity and of regression differences between laboratories. *Annals of Clinical Biochemistry*, **33**: 55–58.

Bilezikian J.P., Raisz L.G. and Rodan G.A. (eds) (2002) *Principles of Bone Biology*, 2nd edition. San Diego: Academic Press Inc.

Christenson R.H. (1997) Biochemical markers of bone metabolism: an overview. *Clinical Biochemistry*, **30**: 573–593.

Cole D.E.C., Webb S. and Chan P.-C. (2007) Update on parathyroid hormone: new tests and new challenges for external quality assessment. *Clinical Biochemistry*, **40**: 585–590.

Horner J. (2006) Basic science of disorders of calcium metabolism and metabolic diseases of bone. *Surgery*, **24**: 215–219.

Ralston S.H. (2005) Structure and metabolism of bone. *Medicine*, **33**: 58–60.

Weaver C.M. and Heaney R.P. (2005) *Calcium in Human Health*. Totowa NJ: Humana Press Inc.

SELF-ASSESSMENT QUESTIONS

1. What are the main forms of calcium in the body?
2. What are the two most important hormones involved in calcium homeostasis?
3. How does PTH affect the blood calcium level?
4. What effect does 1,25-DHCC have on the intestine?
5. Which is the metabolically active vitamin D metabolite found in the kidney?
6. What is the most common cause of hypercalcaemia in hospitalized patients?
7. Which four organs control the blood calcium level?
8. What is the defect in pseudohypoparathyroidism?
9. Give three types of method used to measure calcium in blood.

Control of carbohydrate metabolism

Learning objectives
After studying this chapter you should confidently be able to:

■ **Describe the importance of glucose in many different metabolic pathways.**
Glucose is an important source of energy. Lipolysis is the breakdown of fat and proteolysis is the breakdown of protein. Glucose is stored as glycogen.

■ **Describe the control of blood glucose concentration.**
Insulin has the effect of lowering blood glucose and glucagon has the effect of raising blood glucose. Cortisol and growth hormone also increases blood glucose concentration. Hypoglycaemia occurs when the blood glucose level falls below 2.2 mmol l^{-1}.

■ **Describe the major features of diabetes mellitus.**
The most important disorder of glucose metabolism is diabetes mellitus. In diabetes mellitus the cells cannot take up glucose despite high blood levels. Insulin-dependent diabetes mellitus usually occurs in younger people (type I diabetes). Insulin-independent diabetes mellitus usually occurs in older people (type II diabetes).

■ **Outline the methods used to assess disorders of glucose homeostasis.**
C-peptide levels in the blood reflect the level of insulin in the blood. Most glucose methods use an enzyme to breakdown glucose and develop a coloured product. High glucose concentrations in the blood cause the glycation of proteins and the measurement of glycated proteins gives an indication of the average glucose level in the blood over the previous few weeks or months.

Everything we do requires energy, from sitting to walking and running, even sleeping. Our energy requirement at any particular time depends on the level of activity in which we are engaged. We all take in food, which we process into the material we use to make the energy needed to live. If we eat to excess (as most people on a typical western diet do) we lay down stores of high-energy compounds ready for use at a later time. Ultimately, the fuel we burn in our cells to give energy for life is glucose, which is derived from our diet. Glucose levels in the blood are controlled within reasonably close limits by a complicated interaction of hormones. If we eat large amounts of sweet foods such as chocolate, the glucose absorbed raises the blood concentration, which then is brought back to its original level within a couple of hours. If we go without food for a prolonged time, our stores are broken down to release glucose, which maintains the blood concentration to match the body's requirements. In this chapter we shall discuss the inter-relationship of carbohydrate and lipid metabolism by studying the major hormones controlling the blood glucose concentration. Also, we shall see how a breakdown of this control mechanism leads to disease and how the clinical biochemistry laboratory is involved in aiding the diagnosis of the more common disorders of carbohydrate metabolism.

9.1 GLUCOSE HOMEOSTASIS

Glucose homeostasis is a complicated interaction of metabolic pathways, regulated by a complex web of hormones acting on a number of different tissues and cells. These processes either increase or decrease the blood glucose concentration but they work together in order to maintain an optimal level. Here a brief overview is presented, with an outline of the processes involved shown in *Fig. 9.1.*

   Glucose is derived from carbohydrates taken in the diet. Carbohydrate is digested to the simple sugars: glucose, fructose and galactose. These sugars are absorbed in the intestine and transported to the liver via the portal vein.

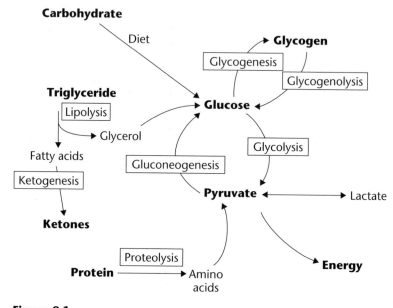

Figure 9.1
Overview of the different mechanisms involved in maintaining the blood glucose concentration within the reference range. These pathways are controlled by a number of hormones, the two most important being insulin and glucagon.

Box 9.1 The pancreas

Special clusters, or islets, scattered through the pancreas were first described by Paul Langerhans in 1869. By 1900 it had been recognized that the β cells in these pancreatic islets were damaged in people dying from diabetes. In 1921 Frederick Banting and his assistant Charles Best showed that the symptoms of diabetes mellitus could be reversed by injecting an extract of islet tissue, and they called this insulin.

In the liver, fructose and galactose can be converted into glucose. Rising levels of glucose in the blood stimulate the release of **insulin** from the β **cells** of the **islets of Langerhans** in the pancreas (see *Box 9.1*). Insulin is the only hormone that reduces blood glucose levels, and it does this by activating the glucose transport mechanisms and glucose-utilizing metabolic pathways in different tissues of the body. Insulin also downregulates glucose-forming pathways. The effects of insulin are given below:

- Stimulates the uptake of glucose by muscle and adipose tissue;
- Stimulates glycolysis;
- Stimulates glycogenesis;
- Stimulates protein synthesis;
- Inhibits gluconeogenesis;
- Inhibits lipolysis;
- Inhibits ketogenesis;
- Inhibits proteolysis.

After a meal, when plenty of glucose is available, insulin is released from the pancreas causing glucose to be used by various metabolic pathways found in a number of different tissues. The pathways that utilize glucose, thereby reducing the blood concentration, are found in many tissues, the most important being the liver, muscle and adipose tissue. The breakdown of glucose by glycolysis and subsequent linkage with the citric acid cycle provides energy in many tissues throughout the body. In the liver, glucose is used to synthesize glycogen, which is then broken down to release glucose in times of need. In muscle, glycogen is also synthesized but acts as a store of energy for use by the muscle tissue when required. In adipose tissue glucose can be processed to form triglyceride and is stored as fat.

When the blood glucose concentration falls, insulin release from the pancreas is also reduced. Low glucose concentrations stimulate the release of **glucagon** from the α **cells** of the islets of Langerhans in the pancreas. Glucagon has the opposite action to insulin, in that it increases the blood glucose concentration. As insulin levels fall and glucagon levels rise, the glucose-utilizing metabolic pathways are switched off and pathways which synthesize glucose are activated. The most important of these pathways are **glycogenolysis, gluconeogenesis, lipolysis** and **proteolysis**.

- Glycogenolysis is the breaking down of glycogen to release glucose. In the liver the glucose is released into the blood stream to raise the glucose concentration, whilst in muscle released glucose is used to provide energy for the muscle cell.

- Gluconeogenesis is the creation of glucose from glycerol (from the breakdown of lipid) or glucogenic amino acids. Most amino acids can be converted to glucose.
- Lipolysis is the breakdown of adipose tissue releasing triglycerides and glycerol that are used to generate energy. Glycerol can itself be converted into glucose. When glucose levels drop to very low levels as a result of starvation or disease, lipolysis is an important source of energy.
- Proteolysis is the breakdown of protein to amino acids that are then used to produce energy.

Many other hormones have a lesser effect on glucose homeostasis, with cortisol, growth hormone, adrenaline and thyroxine being the more important. In health the effect of these hormones is subtle but in pathological conditions where an excess of hormone is present, their effect on glucose concentration can be pronounced, leading to abnormal levels of glucose in the blood.

9.2 INSULIN

Insulin is synthesized in the β cells of the islets of Langerhans and is a protein hormone composed of 51 amino acids (molecular weight 6 kDa). There are two polypeptide chains, an A chain and a B chain, that are joined by two disulphide bonds. Insulin is initially synthesized as preproinsulin, a protein of about 100 amino acids. Preproinsulin is cleaved to generate proinsulin, which is then packaged into storage granules. When insulin is required, proinsulin is further cleaved to give two molecules: C-peptide (molecular weight 3.6 kDa) and insulin, which is then secreted from the cell (see *Box 9.2*).

Box 9.2 Insulin

The American biochemist John Abel crystallized insulin in 1926, the amino acid sequence was deduced by Frederick Sanger in the early 1950s, and the detailed structure was determined in 1972, using X-ray diffraction techniques, by Dorothy Hodgkin.

9.3 DISORDERS OF CARBOHYDRATE METABOLISM

Disorders of glucose metabolism arise from a breakdown in the control mechanisms that regulate glucose concentration in blood, resulting in hyperglycaemia or hypoglycaemia. The reference range for glucose is based on a fasting blood sample, because after food the blood concentration may be highly variable.

Hyperglycaemia

The most important cause of inappropriate hyperglycaemia seen in the clinical laboratory is diabetes mellitus. Blood samples are usually from known patients attending diabetic clinics, although urgent tests are sometimes required to help in the diagnosis of newly presenting diabetics. The symptoms of hyperglycaemia include lassitude, weight loss, polyuria and polydipsia.

Diabetes mellitus

Diabetes mellitus is characterized by the lack, or relative lack of insulin. This has the effect of increasing blood glucose levels as uptake of glucose by cells is inhibited, resulting in glucose deficiency within the cells despite an abundance of glucose outside the cell; this is often called 'starvation amidst a sea of plenty'. Metabolic events within the cell are those seen in cases of starvation. Developing diabetes is characterized by excessive thirst (**polydipsia**) and excess urination (**polyuria**). These symptoms can be attributed to the high levels of glucose in the blood. As glucose levels in the blood gradually rise they eventually exceed the renal threshold for glucose. This happens when the concentration exceeds approximately 10 mmol l^{-1} and results in glucose appearing in the urine. Glucose has strong osmotic activity and acts as an osmotic diuretic, causing an excess of water to be lost in the urine and giving rise to the symptoms of polyuria. In order to replace water, greater amounts of fluid are drunk in order to quench the feeling of thirst, giving the symptoms of polydipsia (see *Box 9.3*).

Box 9.3 Diabetes

It is believed that diabetes was recognized 2500 years ago. The Indians described an illness in 600 BC characterized by excessive thirst and the production of large amounts of sweet urine, and in 500 BC the Egyptians described a similar condition associated with excessive thirst and urination. In the first century AD the Greeks used the word 'diabetes' (meaning to run through a siphon) to describe the condition of excessive urine production where 'the flesh melted down into urine'. In 1674 the English physician Thomas Willis added the word 'mellitus' (the Latin word for honey) to distinguish between this condition and other causes of excessive urine production.

Osmotic diuresis not only causes the loss of water but also of sodium and potassium ions, leading to a gradual depletion of these ions from the body. Diabetes mellitus can be classified into the following:

- Insulin-dependent diabetes mellitus (IDDM); this used to be called type I diabetes mellitus or juvenile-onset diabetes;
- Non-insulin-dependent diabetes mellitus (NIDDM); this used to be called type II diabetes mellitus or adult-onset diabetes;
- Secondary diabetes mellitus.

IDDM is an autoimmune disease resulting in the destruction of insulin-producing cells in the pancreas. It is thought that an environmental trigger, such as a viral infection or a factor involved in neonatal feeding, initiates the disease in those who have a genetic predisposition. Insulin levels gradually drop as the pancreatic β cells are destroyed, until ultimately there is an absolute lack of insulin. None of the metabolic events dependent on insulin can occur and without urgent medical treatment and replacement of insulin the patient will die. These patients need life-long insulin replacement in order to lead a near-normal lifestyle. IDDM usually occurs in the young patient, with a peak between 9 and 14 years, but can occur at any age and accounts for approximately 15% of diabetics.

The remaining 85% of diabetics suffer from NIDDM, which usually occurs between 40 and 80 years but, like IDDM, can present at any age. With NIDDM, symptoms result from the insulin receptor on the cell surface becoming defective, either in terms of number or reduced activity. The insulin message is not carried into the cell efficiently, causing insulin-dependent metabolism to be understimulated. The insulin concentration in these patients is usually normal or high. As obesity is an associated factor in developing NIDDM, often the condition is controlled by diet.

Secondary diabetes mellitus is seen in a number of other conditions such as pancreatic disease or other endocrine disorders where the action of the hormone involved antagonizes the action of insulin, for example in Cushing's syndrome where there is an inappropriate high level of cortisol in the blood.

Complications of diabetes mellitus

Persistent hyperglycaemia leads to the many complications seen in diabetic patients. These complications arise as a result of chemical reactions between glucose and proteins in the body, causing the formation of a **glycated protein**. Glycated proteins associated with blood vessels produce abnormalities in the wall of the blood vessel leading to **microangiopathy**. Changes in blood vessel structure result in the leaking of blood into surrounding tissue spaces and further glycosylation of tissue proteins. Other organs are damaged, such as the eye (leading to **retinopathy**), the kidney (leading to **nephropathy**) and nervous tissue (leading to **neuropathy**). Diabetic patients are also at higher risk of coronary heart disease, perhaps as a result of high lipid levels found in the blood (see *Box 9.4*).

Box 9.4 Cost of diabetes

The prevalence of diabetes has been rising rapidly, with a doubling of the number of people diagnosed with diabetes. In America this went from 8 million people in 1995 to 15.8 million people in 2005. This represents 7% of the total population and 38% of the population over 65 years diagnosed with diabetes. It is estimated that there may be a further 6.2 million undiagnosed cases of diabetes.

Hypoglycaemia

Symptoms of hypoglycaemia include sweating, shaking, nausea, weakness and tachycardia. These symptoms are associated with adrenalin release stimulated by the low glucose concentration. If left untreated and if the blood glucose concentration continues to fall to below 1.0 mmol l^{-1}, coma ensues followed by death.

Hypoglycaemia is usually defined as having a blood glucose concentration lower than 2.5 mmol l^{-1} and can be seen in a wide range of conditions including liver disease, endocrine disease and inborn errors of metabolism. The low glucose concentration found in the blood can be due to:

■ An inability to synthesize sufficient glucose to meet demands;
■ An excessive utilization of glucose;
■ Insufficient glucose intake.

The first two causes listed above are due to a loss of control and regulation of glucose homeostasis. In the first case, an inability to synthesize sufficient glucose is associated with liver disease and some inborn errors of metabolism. The liver is the major organ where glucose is synthesized and released into the blood, and diseases of the liver can reduce metabolic processes to a level where the glucose concentration cannot be sustained. Inborn errors of metabolism which lead to hypoglycaemia are those that have a key enzyme missing from the glucogenic metabolic pathway, preventing the formation of glucose. Some examples of such inborn errors are shown in *Table 9.1*.

Table 9.1 Some inborn errors of metabolism associated with hypoglycaemia and the associated enzyme deficiency

Inborn error of metabolism	Deficient enzyme
Galactosaemia	Galactokinase
Glycogen storage disease type I (von Gierke's disease)	Glucose-6-phosphatase
Glycogen storage disease type VI (Hers' disease)	Hepatic phosphorylase
Hereditary fructose intolerance	Fructose-1-phosphate aldolase

Hypoglycaemia resulting from an insufficient metabolic production of glucose is also seen in the rare condition where there is a lack of cortisol (Addison's disease). In this condition the glucogenic actions of cortisol are absent, resulting in hypoglycaemia.

There are a number of conditions where there is an excessive utilization of glucose, which has the effect of lowering blood glucose. If this is unchecked by normal metabolic control, hypoglycaemia develops. Insulin is the major hormone involved in lowering glucose concentrations, and when there is an inappropriate excess of insulin in the blood, glucose is rapidly taken up by cells and used in the glycolytic metabolic pathways, leading to hypoglycaemia. This is the situation in those patients with an **insulinoma** (a usually benign tumour secreting insulin) and in diabetics who have received too much insulin.

Reactive hypoglycaemia is a condition where glucose levels drop to hypoglycaemic levels after food, often a large meal, or after ingesting large quantities of alcohol. The glucose concentration returns to normal levels later.

9.4 THE INVESTIGATION OF GLUCOSE DISORDERS

In the laboratory, investigation of glucose usually involves the measurement of glucose but can also include the measurement of insulin, C-peptide and other hormones such as cortisol. Markers of diabetic control are widely measured on patients attending the diabetic clinic to monitor the effectiveness of the insulin given and to adjust the dose if necessary. These markers include glycated haemoglobin and fructosamine.

Glucose

Glucose is measured on plasma or whole blood that has been taken into sample tubes containing fluoride to prevent glycolysis, thus preserving glucose in the sample. Blood samples should be taken after the patient has fasted overnight (a fasting sample) although a random sample can be used in emergency situations. Glucose can be measured on venous blood or capillary blood taken from a finger prick. Capillary blood glucose levels are slightly higher than venous glucose levels. *Table 9.2* shows glucose levels that may indicate diabetes in different types of blood sample.

With respect to the investigation of diabetes, two fasting blood samples with a glucose concentration equal to or greater than 8.0 mmol l^{-1} is

Table 9.2 Glucose concentrations which suggest diabetes mellitus for different types of blood sample according to World Health Organization criteria

Sample type	Glucose concentration if diabetic (mmol l^{-1})
Fasting venous blood	≥8.0
Random venous blood	≥10.0
Random capillary blood	≥11.1
Random venous plasma	≥11.1
Random capillary plasma	≥12.2

diagnostic of diabetes, with a borderline result being a concentration between 6.0 and 8.0 mmol l^{-1}.

In order to further clarify borderline results, a glucose tolerance test can be performed on the patient. The patient fasts overnight and a blood sample is taken to measure the fasting glucose concentration. Then the patient drinks a solution containing 75 g of glucose, often mixed with a flavouring of some kind. Blood is taken every 30 minutes for 2 hours and the glucose concentration is measured in each sample. A typical diabetic response and a normal response are shown in *Fig. 9.2*. An inappropriate insulin response to the glucose load will result in a prolonged elevation of blood glucose. A level greater than 11.1 mmol l^{-1} at 2 hours is diagnostic of diabetes.

Urine samples are used to screen for diabetes mellitus as part of health checks and during hospital admissions, and by diabetic patients as an aid

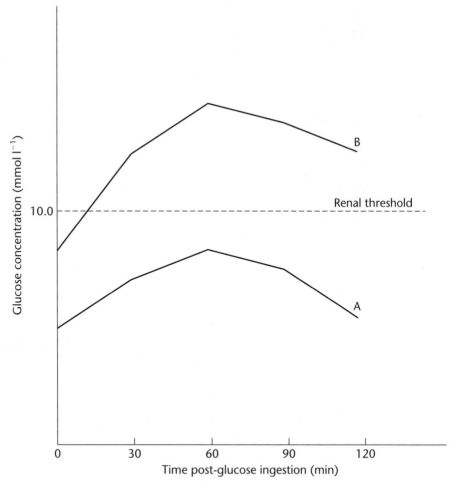

Figure 9.2
Responses to a glucose tolerance test: A, a normal response; and B, a diabetic response.

to monitoring their insulin dose. Any glucose detected indicates that the renal threshold has been exceeded and the blood glucose has risen above 10 mmol l^{-1}.

Methods for measurement of glucose

Glucose is commonly measured using an enzyme to convert the glucose to a product that can be easily detected. Common enzymes used are glucose oxidase, glucose dehydrogenase and hexokinase. Glucose oxidase converts glucose, in the presence of oxygen, to gluconolactone and hydrogen peroxide:

$$\text{Glucose} + O_2 \xrightarrow{\text{Glucose oxidase}} \text{Gluconolactone} + H_2O_2$$

Hydrogen peroxide can be converted to water and oxygen by the action of the enzyme peroxidase. A chromogenic oxygen acceptor (the reduced form) captures the released oxygen (now the oxidized form), and this allows quantitation of the glucose. The oxygen acceptor is usually a non-coloured substance that becomes coloured when oxidized.

$$\underset{\text{(colourless)}}{H_2O_2 + o\text{-Dianisidine}} \xrightarrow{\text{Peroxidase}} \underset{\text{(coloured)}}{\text{Oxidized } o\text{-dianisidine} + H_2O}$$

A number of compounds can interfere with peroxidase, especially in urine samples, giving false low results. These problems can be overcome using the enzyme glucose dehydrogenase, which works on the principle shown below:

$$\text{Glucose} + NAD^+ \xrightarrow{\text{Glucose dehydrogenase}} \text{Glucono-}\delta\text{-lactone} + NADH + H^+$$

The amount of reduced nicotinamide adenine dinucleotide (NADH) produced is proportional to the concentration of glucose in the sample. The production of NADH is monitored by an increasing absorbance at 340 nm.

Methods using hexokinase produce glucose-6-phosphate, which is used as a substrate with NAD$^+$ in a second enzyme reaction using glucose-6-phosphate dehydrogenase. NADH is produced in proportion to the glucose concentration in the sample.

$$\text{Glucose} + ATP \xrightarrow{\text{Hexokinase}} \text{Glucose-6-phosphate} + ADP$$

$$\text{Glucose-6-phosphate} + NAD^+ \xrightarrow{\text{G-6-P dehydrogenase}}$$
$$\text{6-Phosphogluconate} + ADH + H^+$$

A number of electrochemical methods which also use enzymes are available for measuring glucose. One example is the use of an oxygen electrode that measures oxygen consumption after adding glucose oxidase to a sample. Other electrochemical methods measure the hydrogen peroxide produced by glucose oxidase, by oxidation of hydrogen peroxide at an electrode surface.

The home monitoring of glucose by diabetics is performed using 'dipsticks' that have glucose oxidase, peroxidase and a chromogen impregnated in a small absorbent pad. The reagents are dried and when a drop of blood is dropped on the test area, a colour change is seen, which is proportional to the concentration of glucose in the sample. If performed well and following the manufacturer's instructions, reasonably reliable results can be achieved. In recent years a number of electrochemical devices have become available for home monitoring of glucose. One such device is shaped like a pen; a drop of blood is placed on the electrode 'nib' and a reading is given on the stem of the pen.

Insulin

Plasma insulin concentrations are useful in the investigation of hypoglycaemia and the investigation of an insulinoma. Methods for measuring insulin are based on sandwich immunoassay techniques employing labelled antibodies.

C-peptide

Measurement of C-peptide is useful in assessing the production of natural insulin. When insulin is secreted by the pancreas, there is an equimolar release of C-peptide. This allows hyperglycaemia due to insulinoma, with a high C-peptide, to be differentiated from hyperglycaemia, due to administration of insulin, with a low C-peptide. Measurement is by an immunoassay.

Glycated proteins

Glycated (sometimes called glycosylated) haemoglobin occurs as a result of the reaction of glucose with haemoglobin (Hb). In adults 97% of haemoglobin is HbA. A number of minor variants of HbA exist, referred to as HbA_{1a}, HbA_{1b} and HbA_{1c}, collectively called HbA_1, with HbA_{1c} being the major fraction. The formation of glycated haemoglobin occurs over the lifespan of the erythrocyte, averaging 120 days. The amount of total HbA_1 depends on the average glucose concentration over the previous 2 or 3 months. Short-term fluctuations in the glucose concentration do not affect the level of glycated haemoglobin. The value of glycated haemoglobin is in the medium-term assessment of diabetic control and as an aid to patient management. Values are reported as percentages of total blood haemoglobin with the following reference ranges:

HbA_1	5.0–8.0%
HbA_{1c}	3.0–6.0%

Other proteins are also glycated by glucose and the extent of the glycation can be assessed by measuring fructosamine, which is the ketoamine produced by glycation. The major protein in plasma is albumin which has a half-life of about 19 days in blood. Glycated albumin is the major contributor in fructosamine measurements, and measuring this gives an indication of glucose control over the previous 3 weeks.

Glycated proteins are measured using a range of techniques including ion-exchange chromatography, high-performance liquid chromatography (HPLC), affinity chromatography, electrophoresis, isoelectric focusing and immunoassay.

SUGGESTED FURTHER READING

In addition to relevant chapters in the text books cited in Chapters 1 and 5, the following references are recommended.

Kahn R. (2007) *Annual Review of Diabetes.* American Diabetes Association.

Savoca R., Jaworek B. and Huber A.R. (2006) New "plasma referenced" POCT glucose monitoring systems – are they suitable for glucose monitoring and diagnosis of diabetes? *Clinica Chimica Acta,* **372**: 199–201.

Winter W.E. and Signorino M.R. (2002) *Diabetes Mellitus: Pathophysiology, Etiologies, Complications, Management, and Laboratory Evaluation.* Washington, DC: American Association for Clinical Chemistry.

SELF-ASSESSMENT QUESTIONS

1. What are the major two hormones that control blood levels of glucose?
2. In which two important tissues does insulin stimulate glucose uptake?
3. What two symptoms are seen in a patient developing diabetes mellitus?
4. Describe the main categories of diabetes mellitus.
5. What is the renal threshold for glucose in most people?
6. Does von Gierke's disease cause hyper- or hypoglycaemia?
7. How should the patient be prepared before investigating glucose homeostasis?
8. How can proteins be useful in assessing glucose homeostasis?
9. Would you expect high or low blood glucose in a patient with an insulinoma?
10. Name four enzymes that use glucose as a substrate and have been used in the measurement of glucose.

Enzymes

In this section we shall look at how diseases which affect the systems which **process** material can be investigated in the clinical biochemistry laboratory. Enzymes are used to process many different substrates to turn them into a product. In this chapter we shall see how the presence of enzymes in the plasma can be used to indicate disease of particular organs, and in the following chapter we shall see how abnormalities of particular enzymes lead to other types of disease.

Enzymes are proteins which are folded in a particular manner, allowing them to combine with a specific substrate and convert it into a product, which may be a slightly altered form of the substrate or quite different from the substrate. Thus, an enzyme is a **biological catalyst** and is responsible for the processing and synthesis of many molecules within a cell. Life requires the action of many enzymes to provide the building blocks to make new cells, to provide energy in order to live, and to maintain health.

In a cell many enzymes are linked together to form a metabolic pathway, with the product from the first enzyme reaction acting as the substrate for the second enzyme, which then in turn forms a second product which acts as the substrate for the third enzyme and so on. Different cells in different tissues will have different metabolic pathways running and so there are different enzymes present in these various tissues. For example, muscle is rich in the enzyme creatine kinase, whereas the liver cells have little creatine kinase but are rich in the enzyme aspartate transaminase. By understanding which enzymes are present in high concentrations in different tissues, enzymes can be used to look for **tissue damage**. If an enzyme which should be present in a cell within a particular tissue is found in high levels in the blood, then tissue damage may have occurred. In this chapter we shall study clinically important enzymes which can be measured in blood and reflect tissue damage, and we shall discuss the clinical significance of enzyme measurements (see *Box 10.1*).

Box 10.1 Enzymes

The German organic chemist Eduard Buchner showed, in 1897, that fermentation did not require living cells. He made an extract from yeast cells, which he called zymase. Sir Arthur Harden went on to demonstrate that zymase was a mixture of enzymes, where each enzyme catalysed one step in the conversion of sugar to ethanol. In 1907 and 1929, Buchner and then Harden were awarded the Nobel Prize for Chemistry for their work. Later in the 20th century John Northrop crystallized an enzyme and showed it to be a protein. He did this using urease and then went on to study other enzymes.

Most enzymes are found within cells and they may act on particular substrates that are specific to that cell or on a substrate common to many different types of cell. Some enzymes are synthesized within cells and are secreted to work either in the blood or in the gut. Examples of enzymes that are designed to function in the blood are the enzymes involved in the blood clotting process. The enzymes of digestion are secreted into the gut where food is the substrate.

Within the cell there are two main regions where enzymes are located: in the **cytosol** and bound to **membranes** of cell organelles. If the cell is damaged, at first cytosolic enzymes leak into the surrounding tissue fluid, whilst those enzymes bound to membranes within the cell remain in the cell. When cells become more damaged or are destroyed, both cytosolic and membrane-bound enzymes are released into the surrounding tissue fluid. Cells can be easily damaged by many different factors, probably the most common being **hypoxia** (low oxygen level). Mild hypoxia renders the cell membrane leaky, allowing the loss of cytosolic enzymes; this damage is reversible. *Table 10.1* lists the more important causes of cell damage that allow the release of intracellular contents (see *Box 10.2*).

Table 10.1 Some causes and examples of cell damage and death

Hypoxia	Myocardial infarction
Toxic substances	Drugs, heavy metals, alcohol abuse
Infections	Viral hepatitis
Trauma	Crush injuries
Immune destruction	Autoimmune disease

Box 10.2 Enzyme structure and activity

Christian Anfinsen showed that the three-dimensional shape of an enzyme was important for its specific activity towards its substrate. He was awarded a Nobel Prize in 1972 with Stanford Moore and William Stein for their work on the structure of enzymes. Moore and Stein were recognized for their work in developing the first method of analysing amino acids, derived from hydrolysing protein.

10.1 ISOENZYMES AND ISOFORMS

The structure of an enzyme is determined by a particular gene. That enzyme will combine with a specific substrate which is broken down to form a product, and the specificity of the enzyme is determined by the active site. An enzyme in the cell of a different tissue may be coded for by a separate gene but the active site may be very similar. Thus, despite this being a different protein, it has the same enzymatic activity. When two different proteins from different tissues, encoded by different genes, act on the same substrate, these are termed **isoenzymes**. Isoenzymes are synthesized in different cells of different tissues and, although they show the same enzymatic action, they have different physical properties and can therefore be separated using methods such as electrophoresis. Studying isoenzyme patterns in blood allows a more tissue-specific marker to be used in the investigation of tissue damage. A good example of this type of study is the enzyme creatine kinase, found in skeletal muscle, cardiac muscle and brain tissue. Creatine kinase measured in the blood could have arisen from damage to any of these tissues, but by looking at a specific isoenzyme or the isoenzyme pattern, the damaged tissue can be identified. For instance, by measuring the cardiac-specific creatine kinase, a good indication of cardiac damage can be obtained, which is useful in the assessment of myocardial infarction.

Enzyme molecules may undergo structural modifications after they have been synthesized in the cell. These changes are normal modifications and may reflect ageing of the enzyme. Enzyme structure can be modified by the action and binding of other molecules, for example glucose, resulting in a protein with altered physical properties. In other cases the protein chain may lose terminal amino acids, again modifying the enzyme molecule. These changes to the basic enzyme structure are **post-translational modifications**. Enzymes that differ from one another by a post-translational modification are called **isoforms**. Isoenzymes usually arise from different tissues but isoforms are modifications of an isoenzyme and, as such, they arise from the same tissue and may reflect ageing of the enzyme. The longer the enzyme has been in the cell or in the blood, the greater the chance of a post-translational modification taking place. Clinically interesting isoforms of creatine kinase are seen, which can be important in the assessment of cardiac disease.

10.2 CLINICALLY IMPORTANT ENZYMES

The following enzymes are the most frequently measured in the clinical biochemistry laboratory. They are associated with conditions where cellular disruption has led to the release of the enzymes into the surrounding fluid, eventually finding their way into the blood.

Aspartate aminotransferase (AST) and alanine aminotransferase (ALT)

These are probably the most frequently measured enzymes in the clinical biochemistry laboratory. These enzymes are found in most tissues throughout the body but especially in skeletal muscle, cardiac muscle, liver and kidney. AST has two isoenzymes, one being cytoplasmic and the other being bound to mitochondrial membranes. ALT is only found in the cytoplasm. AST is widely measured in the investigation of liver disease and in cases of suspected myocardial infarction. Measurements are not highly specific because many tissues have high levels of AST. Where the disease is known, measurements of AST may be useful in following the progression or treatment of the disease: falling AST levels in the blood would indicate that the treatment is successful and the patient is making a recovery (see *Box 10.3*).

ALT is usually only measured in the investigation of liver disease, although it is also present in many other tissues. ALT or AST are often measured as part of a liver function test profile. Occasionally a laboratory may measure both ALT and AST, as some prognostic indication of liver disease may be obtained. When there is slight damage to the liver cells both AST and ALT will rise at a similar rate, reaching similar levels in the blood.

Box 10.3 Aminotransferases

The aminotransferases are a group of enzymes that catalyse the transfer of an amino group between amino acids and α-oxoacids. AST catalyses the reversible reaction:

$$\text{L-Aspartate} + \alpha\text{-Oxoglutarate} \rightleftharpoons \text{Oxaloacetate} + \text{L-Glutamate}$$

whilst ALT catalyses the reversible reaction:

$$\text{L-Alanine} + \alpha\text{-Oxoglutarate} \rightleftharpoons \text{Pyruvate} + \text{L-Glutamate}$$

This is due to the cytoplasmic enzymes being released from the damaged cell, whilst membrane-bound enzymes are retained by the cell. In the event of greater damage to the cell, membrane-bound enzymes are also released into the surrounding tissue fluid. In liver disease where there is irreversible damage to the liver cells, the membrane-bound AST is also released, causing blood AST levels to rise to a greater extent than the ALT levels. By calculating the ratio of AST to ALT an indication of the severity of liver damage can be obtained.

Creatine kinase (CK)

CK, also known as creatine phosphokinase (CPK), is a dimeric enzyme composed of two protein chains. Each protein chain is either a B chain or an M chain, and these can associate to form three dimers, each dimer being a different isoenzyme. The three isoenzymes of CK are known as CK-MM, CK-MB and CK-BB. Although CK is widely distributed throughout the body, the isoenzymes are found in relatively higher concentrations in some tissues. CK-BB is found in high concentrations in brain tissue, CK-MM is found mainly in skeletal muscle and CK-MB is found in relatively high concentrations in cardiac muscle (see *Box 10.4*).

Box 10.4 Creatine kinase

CK catalyses the reversible phosphorylation of creatine by adenosine triphosphate (ATP):

$$Creatine + ATP \rightleftharpoons Phosphocreatine + Adenosine\ diphosphate$$

In the plasma, CK can be modified by an enzyme, called a carboxypeptidase, which removes the terminal lysine amino acid residue from the CK-M subunit. The enzyme activity of CK is not affected but the loss of the terminal lysine changes the electrophoretic mobility of the enzyme and the modified CK is known as an isoform. CK-MM, which has both terminal lysine residues removed, is known as CK-MM1, whereas the isoform with only one terminal lysine removed is called CK-MM2, and the intact molecule is the CK-MM3 isoform. The clinical significance of different amounts of the isoforms in the blood is doubtful, although interest has been shown in the ratio of CK-MM3 to CK-MM1, which may have a diagnostic value in investigating patients with suspected myocardial infarction.

Total CK measurements are useful in the investigation of muscle disease, and despite its lack of specificity, many laboratories measure total CK levels in the investigation of patients with suspected myocardial infarction.

Lactate dehydrogenase (LDH)

LDH is an important enzyme found throughout the body, comprising five major isoenzymes. The enzyme is a tetrameric molecule made from four subunits, where there are two different types of subunit (H or M). Different numbers of subunits can combine together to form the five different iso-enzymes, as shown below.

Subunits		LDH isoenzyme
HHHH	(H4)	LDH1
HHHM	(H3M)	LDH2
HHMM	(H2M2)	LDH3
HMMM	(H1M3)	LDH4
MMMM	(M4)	LDH5

LDH1 is found predominantly in heart muscle (H subunit) and in red blood cells. This is the most stable isoenzyme and runs the furthest on an electrophoresis strip. In contrast, LDH5, found predominantly in liver and skeletal muscle (M subunit), is the least stable isoenzyme and runs the short-est distance on electrophoresis. LDH isoenzymes are composed of mixtures of the H and M subunits; for example, LDH3 (two H and two M subunits), is found in a variety of tissues such as spleen, lung, endocrine glands and lymph nodes. The analysis of isoenzyme patterns can help in the investiga-tion of myocardial infarction, where elevated levels of LDH1 and LDH2 are found. In health there is more LDH2 than LDH1, but following damage to cardiac muscle, LDH1 is released into the blood causing there to be more LDH1 than LDH2. This is known as a 'flipped LDH isoenzyme pattern'. *Figure 10.1* shows the results of a densitometer scan of LDH isoenzymes separated by electrophoresis: the pattern in (a) is normal, whilst pattern (b) shows elevation of LDH1 relative to the other isoenzymes, giving the flipped pattern (see *Box 10.5*).

The complete analysis of LDH isoenzymes is not often requested, but more commonly a selective substrate is used. 2-oxobutyrate is often used as a specific substrate for LDH1; when using this substrate LDH1 is known as **hydroxybutyrate dehydrogenase** (HBD).

LDH-5 is found predominantly in skeletal muscle and in the liver, and therefore diseases of these tissues will tend to give elevated levels of LDH4 and LDH5.

Box 10.5 Lactate dehydrogenase

LDH catalyses the transfer of a hydrogen ion between lactate and NAD^+:

$$Lactate + NAD^+ \rightleftharpoons Pyruvate + NADH + H^+$$

In the body the reverse reaction is favoured, i.e. pyruvate to lactate.

Alkaline phosphatase

This is the name for a group of enzymes that have maximal activity at a high pH, in the range 9.0–10.5. These enzymes are widely distributed throughout the body and found in many different tissues. The most impor-

(a)

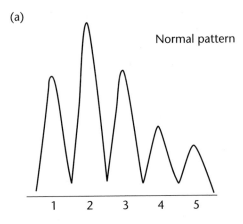

Normal pattern

(b)

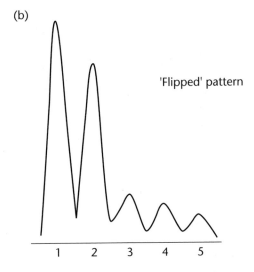

'Flipped' pattern

Figure 10.1
The results of a densitometer scan of LDH isoenzymes separated by electrophoresis. A normal pattern is seen in (a), showing LDH2 to be the most abundant. Pattern (b) shows elevation of LDH1 and LDH2 with a greater rise in LDH1; this is the 'flipped pattern' characteristic of myocardial infarction.

tant tissues where high levels of alkaline phosphatase are found include the liver, bone, placenta and intestine. In the liver, alkaline phosphatase is found in high concentrations in the cells lining the biliary ducts and it is therefore a marker of cholestatic liver disease. The alkaline phosphatase enzymes found in these different tissues are isoenzymes and can be separated by electrophoresis, or individual isoenzymes can be assessed using inhibitors, specific substrates or by heat inactivation of the other isoenzymes. Despite the importance of the isoenzymes, the most frequently requested alkaline phosphatase measurement is the total enzyme activity. This is an easy and rapid assay that would form part of a liver or bone screen. As expected from the above discussion, an elevated alkaline phosphatase level is usually associated with liver or bone disease.

Acid phosphatase

This group of enzymes has maximal activity in the pH range of 5–6. The prostate gland, liver, spleen and red blood cells all contain acid phosphatase enzymes. The greatest source of acid phosphatase is the prostate gland, and it has been in the monitoring of prostate disease that acid phosphatase measurements have been most useful. The prostatic isoenzyme of acid phosphatase is the more clinically useful measurement and, by making use of a specific inhibitor, this prostatic form is easily measured. Traditionally, the inhibitor L-tartrate has been used because of its ability to selectively inhibit the prostatic isoenzyme. Two acid phosphatase measurements are performed, the total and tartrate specific (non-prostatic), with the resulting difference between the measurements being the prostatic acid phosphatase activity. Modern measurements are made using specific immunoassay techniques. High levels are seen in cases of prostate cancer and this enzyme has been used to monitor treatment of the disease, although these days a more specific marker of prostate disease is used, namely prostate-specific antigen (PSA).

An increased level of acid phosphatase can also be due to the tartrate-stable isoenzyme (non-prostatic), which is sometimes seen in patients with bone or liver disease.

γ-Glutamyltransferase (GGT, γ-GT)

GGT is found mainly in the biliary ducts of the liver, in the kidney and pancreas, with the largest amounts being found in the kidney. The most important diagnostic use of GGT measurements, however, is in liver disease. Levels will often mirror those of alkaline phosphatase, with the highest levels being seen in cholestasis. GGT is also found in the hepatocytes where its enzyme activity can be induced by a number of drugs and in particular alcohol. This makes GGT a useful marker of alcohol-induced liver disease and, in particular, liver cirrhosis.

Amylase

Amylase is found in high concentrations in the pancreas and salivary glands where it is secreted to digest complex carbohydrates. Measurements of amylase activity are useful in those patients with acute abdominal pain, to differentiate between patients with acute pancreatitis and those with appendicitis. Patients with acute pancreatitis will have high levels of amylase in their blood.

10.3 ENZYMES AND TISSUE DAMAGE

In the clinical biochemistry laboratory a number of enzymes are measured in order to assess tissue damage to a particular organ. In this section we shall discuss the important enzymes associated with damage to a number of different tissues. The most important organs in which enzyme measurements are clinically important include heart, skeletal muscle, liver and bone.

Cardiac enzymes

The measurement of cardiac-specific enzymes is useful in the diagnosis and assessment of prognosis of **myocardial infarction**. A number of different enzymes have been used, but many suffer from the problem of not being totally tissue specific. For example, AST is present in relatively high concentrations in cardiac muscle cells, but is also present in high concentrations in other tissues such as the liver and kidney. In most modern laboratories the enzyme of choice in assessing myocardial infarction is CK, and a few laboratories also measure LDH.

Myocardial infarction is characterized by a sudden onset of chest pain, although in some patients, particularly elderly patients, the chest pain may be absent. Diagnosis is usually given after characteristic changes on an electrocardiograph are seen, although some patients may not develop these characteristic patterns until some time later. Enzyme measurements give the opportunity to assess the patient for cardiac damage by taking a blood sample. Early diagnosis is essential in this condition, as the sooner treatment can be started, the better the prognosis for the patient. The time at which the blood sample is taken from the patient is critical; if it is taken too early after the onset of symptoms, then there has been insufficient time to allow the enzyme levels in the blood to rise sufficiently to give a meaningful result. If the patient comes into hospital a day or two after the onset of chest pain, then the levels of enzyme in the blood may be dropping and an inappropriate diagnosis could be made. Not only is the timing of the sample important but a knowledge of the kinetics involved in the changes seen in blood levels of the different enzymes released from damaged cardiac tissue is also required. The different enzymes involved have different rates of release from cardiac tissue. For example, CK rises rapidly in the first 18 hours after the onset of chest pain, reaching a maximum level at approximately 24 hours. CK levels then fall rapidly, reaching a normal concentration by day 3. On the other hand, LDH rises more slowly, reaching a maximum level on about day 4, after which the enzyme levels in the blood slowly fall and reach normal levels by day 9 or 10. CK measurements are useful for making a rapid diagnosis if the patient has been brought into hospital soon after suffering chest pain, whereas LDH is a more appropriate enzyme marker when the patient presents some days following the initial chest pain. *Figure 10.2* shows changes in serum concentrations of AST, CK and LDH over time.

New advances are being made with other biochemical markers of cardiac damage, many of which are not enzymes. In recent years much interest has

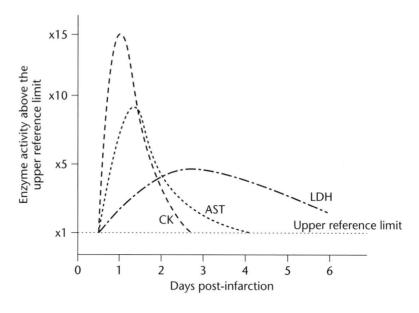

Figure 10.2
The rise and fall of enzyme activity in the blood following a myocardial infarction.
Creatine kinase (CK) rises first and is first to return to normal. Aspartate
aminotransferase (AST) closely follows CK. Lactate dehydrogenase (LDH) is the last
enzyme to peak and takes the longest to return to normal levels.

been shown in muscle proteins called **troponins**. There are three troponin
proteins involved in muscle contraction: **troponin T, toponin C** and
troponin I. Most interest has been shown in the cardiac-specific forms of
troponin T and troponin I, which have high sensitivity and specificity for
differentiating between patients with myocardial infarction and patients
with non-cardiac chest pain.

Liver enzymes

Liver disease can be divided into diseases of the hepatocytes and diseases
involving the biliary tract, or cholestatic disease. Clinical biochemistry laboratories often measure enzymes as part of a liver function test. AST or ALT are
usually measured as an indicator of hepatic damage. Very high levels are found
in the blood in cases of hepatitis and hepatocellular toxicity, such as that
found in an overdose of paracetamol. Alkaline phosphatase, an enzyme associated with cholestasis, may be only slightly raised in cases of hepatitis but is
greatly raised in cholestasis. Cholestasis is a blockage of the biliary ducts,
which can occur within the liver, called intrahepatic cholestasis, or outside the
liver, called extrahepatic cholestasis. The liver enzymes frequently measured
that reflect cholestatic disease are alkaline phosphatase and GGT. These
enzymes are only slightly raised in hepatic disease but can be greatly raised in
cholestatic conditions such as biliary obstruction due to liver tumours, giving

rise to intrahepatic cholestasis, or pancreatic tumours, giving rise to extra-hepatic cholestasis. Liver cirrhosis caused by alcohol abuse is often detected and monitored using GGT. Further discussion on liver disease is given in Chapter 18.

Muscle enzymes

In the clinical biochemistry laboratory CK is measured to give an indication of muscle damage. The majority of CK is found in skeletal muscle and is released in large quantities with damage to that muscle. Other enzymes may also be elevated with muscle damage, such as the transaminases and LDH, but CK is the enzyme of choice. High levels of total CK are found where there has been muscle damage or injury, and even unaccustomed exercise will cause huge amounts of enzyme to be released from the muscle cells into the blood. Muscle disease such as muscular dystrophy will also give elevated CK levels in the blood. It is important to differentiate between skeletal muscle disease or damage and cardiac muscle damage, because both conditions will give an elevated total CK.

Inborn errors of metabolism

Another application for enzyme measurements is in the investigation of an inborn error of metabolism (this subject is discussed fully in Chapter 11). In such conditions the enzyme is not fully active, resulting in a pathological condition called an **inherited metabolic disorder**. As part of an investigation, the activity of the enzyme is measured in blood and sometimes in preparations of cells such as fibroblasts. If both genes are affected (i.e. the patient is homozygous), then there will be very little enzyme activity detected, but if only one gene is affected (i.e. the patient is heterozygous), then approximately 50% of the normal enzyme activity will be observed. Some examples of inherited metabolic disorders and the affected enzyme are given in *Table 10.2*.

Table 10.2 Examples of inborn errors of metabolism and the enzyme affected

Disorder	Enzyme affected
Phenylketonuria	Phenylalanine hydroxylase
Alkaptonuria	Homogentisic acid oxidase
Galactosaemia	Galactokinase or galactose-1-phosphate uridyl transferase
von Gierke's disease	Glucose-6-phosphatase
Tay–Sachs disease	β-N-Acetylglucosaminidase A
Hurler's syndrome	α-L-Iduronidase

10.4 PRINCIPLES OF ENZYME MEASUREMENTS

Enzymes work at an optimum pH, temperature and ionic strength and may also require the presence of a prosthetic group, cofactor or divalent metal ion for maximal activity. These factors must be taken into account when designing a buffer for use in a particular enzyme measurement. In addition, the buffer must contain a substrate for that particular enzyme. Enzyme activity is calculated from the appearance of product or disappearance of substrate. Some methods rely on the use of artificial substrates that yield a coloured product, whereas others rely on the measurement of a cofactor, for example NAD or NADH. The production or utilization of NAD or NADP is easily monitored by measuring the change in absorbance at 340 nm as NADH and NADPH absorb strongly at 340 nm but the oxidized forms do not. The definitions of international units and katels (units of enzyme activity) are given in Chapter 1.

When measuring enzyme activity in blood samples it is important that the method used is optimized, not only in terms of pH, temperature, etc. but also, more importantly, in terms of substrate concentration. The enzyme being measured must obey **zero-order kinetics**, where the enzyme reaction rate is independent of the substrate concentration; the importance of this is described below.

At low substrate concentrations the rate or velocity of an enzyme reaction is dependent on the concentration of substrate [S] (this is the molar concentration). This rate of reaction changes as [S] changes until a maximum rate, called the maximum velocity (V_{max}), is reached. At this point the enzyme is saturated and the enzyme reaction is independent of [S]; this is shown graphically in *Fig. 10.3*. In other words, the enzyme reaction rate is constant no matter how much more substrate is added to the reaction mixture. The concentration of substrate which gives a reaction rate equivalent to half V_{max} is called the Michaelis–Menten constant (K_m). This is shown in *Fig. 10.3*.

Where the reaction is proportional to the substrate concentration, i.e. when the enzyme is not saturated, the enzyme reaction is said to be of first order kinetics. In a situation of excess substrate, the enzyme is saturated and the reaction rate is constant; at this point the enzyme reaction is said to be of zero order kinetics, i.e. independent of the substrate concentration. This is demonstrated in *Fig. 10.4*. When the enzyme reaction rate is constant, the amount of product formed is related to the amount of enzyme present in the sample. A sample with a large amount of enzyme present will turn over more substrate in a given time than a sample with a lower amount of enzyme; in other words, there is greater enzyme activity present in the sample with more enzyme molecules.

Enzyme assays should be optimized with sufficient substrate so that the reaction will have zero-order kinetics (as a rule of thumb, the substrate concentration should be 10 times more than the K_m for that enzyme). In this situation the rate of product formation is constant over time, as seen in *Fig. 10.5a*. If insufficient substrate is present in the tube then the reaction will begin to show first-order kinetics, i.e. the reaction rate is dependent on [S]. As the reaction proceeds, substrate is depleted and the reaction rate

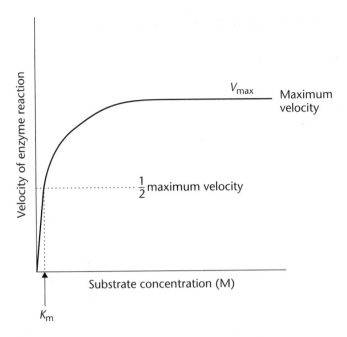

Figure 10.3
Graph to show the velocity of enzyme reaction against substrate concentration. At V_{max} the enzyme is saturated and the reaction obeys zero-order kinetics. The Michaelis–Menten constant (K_m) is the concentration of substrate at half V_{max}.

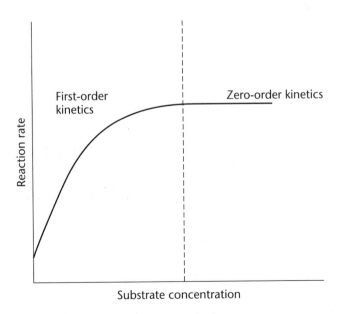

Figure 10.4
Graph to show the difference between first- and zero-order kinetics.

(a)

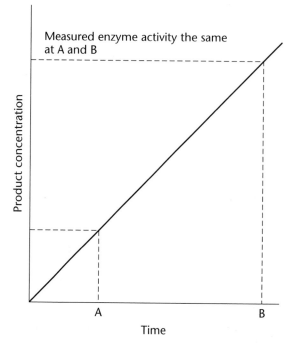

Constant rate=zero-order kinetics

Measured enzyme activity the same at A and B

Product concentration

Time

A

B

(b)

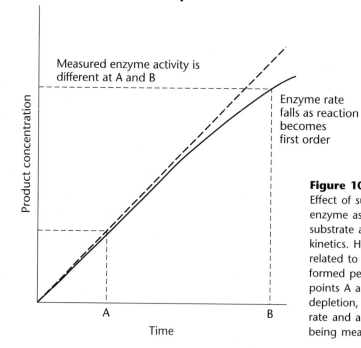

Substrate depletion

Measured enzyme activity is different at A and B

Enzyme rate falls as reaction becomes first order

Product concentration

Time

A

B

Figure 10.5
Effect of substrate depletion on an enzyme assay. In (a) there is excess substrate and therefore zero-order kinetics. Here the enzyme activity, as related to the amount of product formed per unit of time, is the same at points A and B. In (b) there is substrate depletion, resulting in a fall in reaction rate and a different enzyme activity being measured at A and B.

changes over time, leading to an underestimation of the enzyme activity, as shown in *Fig. 10.5b*. Samples with very high levels of enzyme may rapidly deplete the available substrate in the reaction tube, again leading to a loss of zero-order kinetics and an underestimation of the enzyme activity.

Enzyme activity is calculated from the change in absorbance due to the accumulation of product. This can be measured as the difference in absorbance over a defined time period or by measuring the rate of change in absorbance. Most manual techniques measure the difference in absorbance over a given time period. This is known as an **end-point** determination. This is quick and easy but careful timing must be used. Most analytical instrumentation measures the enzyme activity in a blood sample using a **kinetic** method. Here the change in absorbance is constantly monitored and the slope of absorbance change versus time gives the enzyme activity. It is easy for a computer to check that the slope of absorbance change is linear; if the substrate becomes depleted the slope loses linearity and an underestimation of the enzyme activity will be made.

Measurement of enzyme activity is the usual way of assessing the amount of enzyme present in the blood, but in some instances enzymes can be measured by an immunoassay. This approach is usually applied to isoenzymes where an involved separation by electrophoresis is undesirable. When using these types of assay it is not the activity of the enzyme that is being measured but the concentration of protein. This type of measurement is known as a **mass measurement**.

10.5 BIOSENSORS

Enzymes have been used extensively in developing new technology, known as biosensors, for rapid testing for **point-of-care** applications. A biosensor is the integration of a biological molecule with a transducer and an electrical measurement system. The biological molecule gives specificity to the system, which responds to specific biological interactions on the surface of the transducer. The transducer converts the biological interaction into a measurable electrical signal. *Figure 10.6* shows a biosensor with different types of biological molecule that have been used on the surface of the sensor, and also different types of transducer. The most successful biosensor produced so far is the glucose sensor often used for point-of-care testing. This biosensor uses the enzyme glucose oxidase immobilized on the sensor surface. Glucose oxidase breaks down glucose to gluconolactone and hydrogen peroxide, which is electrochemically oxidized by the electrode to generate a current. The meter gives a direct readout of the glucose concentration in the sample, often in less than a minute. Most glucose meters will measure the glucose concentration in a small drop of blood from a finger prick. Many hospitals use glucose meters on the wards and outpatient departments for rapid glucose measurements, and the clinical biochemistry laboratory (in the UK) often takes responsibility for training staff in the use of the instrumentation and maintenance of quality assurance protocols. Examples of

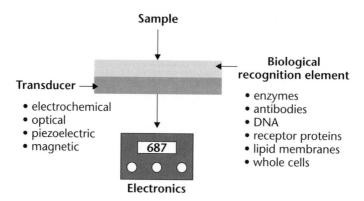

Figure 10.6
Schematic diagram of a biosensor, showing the common type of biological molecule and detection technologies.

other enzyme-based biosensors include sensors for the rapid measurement of cholesterol, urea, lactate and alcohol.

SUGGESTED FURTHER READING

In addition to relevant chapters in the text books cited in Chapter 1 the following references are recommended.

Bugg T. (2004) *Introduction to Enzyme and Coenzyme Chemistry*, 2nd edition. Oxford: Blackwell Publishing.

Holstege A., Zolinski P., Woidy L. and Permanetter W. (2007) The patient with unexplained elevated serum liver enzymes. *Best Practice & Research Clinical Gastroenterology*, **21**: 535–550.

Yang Z. and Min Zhou D. (2006) Cardiac markers and their point-of-care testing for diagnosis of acute myocardial infarction. *Clinical Biochemistry*, **39**: 771–780.

SELF-ASSESSMENT QUESTIONS

1. Which intracellular enzymes are lost through a leaky membrane?
2. What are the main isoenzymes of creatine kinase?
3. What is an enzyme isoform?
4. How many isoenzymes of LDH are there?
5. Which two important tissues give rise to elevated alkaline phosphatase levels when diseased?
6. Which enzyme is useful for monitoring alcoholics?

7. Following a myocardial infarction, which enzyme becomes elevated in the blood first?
8. Is AST a marker of hepatic or cholestatic disease?
9. Why are zero-order kinetics important in measuring enzyme activity in blood?
10. Which two techniques are used for calculating enzyme activity?

Inborn errors of metabolism

Learning objectives
After studying this chapter you should confidently be able to:

■ **Describe the origin of an inborn error of metabolism.**
An inborn error of metabolism arises from a damaged gene, which generally gives rise to an abnormal enzyme. Inborn errors of metabolism can affect many different biochemical pathways. Inborn errors of metabolism are inherited through the autosomes or sex chromosomes.

■ **Explain the inheritance patterns of inborn errors of metabolism.**
Inherited disease can be recessive or dominant in its expression. A heterozygote will have both a normal and an abnormal allele, and a homozygote will have two alleles the same on each chromosome. A recessive disease is only seen in the homozygote expression of abnormal genes. Dominant expression is seen whenever an abnormal gene is inherited.

■ **Outline the laboratory involvement in the investigation of a suspected inborn error of metabolism.**
Screening is used to detect the presence of abnormal genes in the absence of disease symptoms. Prenatal diagnosis is the investigation for an inborn error of metabolism in an unborn child. Newborn babies are routinely screened for PKU and congenital hypothyroidism. PKU is an autosomal recessive disease giving elevated levels of phenylalanine. Cystic fibrosis is the most common genetic disease in the UK.

The day-to-day running of the cell machinery is conducted through the intricate workings of a highly complex web of metabolic pathways. Some cells will perform particular jobs, whilst other cells in different organs will perform a different task. For example, a liver cell has many metabolic pathways through which it processes nutrients thereby producing energy, forming storage material or breaking down unwanted material and excreting it to the outside world. Enzymes are vital for the operation of these metabolic pathways, which in turn can be controlled by hormone action on the cell by activating and inactivating particular enzymes in the pathway.

It is the enzyme that converts a particular substrate to a product and, in a metabolic pathway, this product is a substrate for a second enzyme and so on. In a cell the enzyme is manufactured from its genetic template stored within the DNA as a gene. This genetic template is the same in every cell. In some circumstances the genetic material in a particular cell can be damaged and the gene for a particular enzyme will be slightly altered. In normal circumstances, in a healthy adult this would go unnoticed, as all the surrounding cells would be making the proper enzyme. However, if the cell were a gamete, the mutated gene could be carried to the next generation where all the cells would carry the code for the mutated enzyme and those cells which expressed that gene would make a mutated enzyme. If the mutation caused an alteration at a critical part of the molecule, such as the active site, the enzyme could have reduced or even no enzymatic activity. This would lead to an impairment or blockage of the metabolic pathway which the enzyme served. Typically this could lead to a number of biochemical changes, which would be observed in a patient who displayed a defective enzyme (see *Box 11.1*).

Inborn errors of metabolism (IBEM) involve the **inheritance** of an abnormal gene from one or both parents. Traditionally these have been associated with defects in enzymes and there are examples from a wide range of different metabolic pathways. Today, defects in other types of protein have been recognized, a good example being cystic fibrosis where the defective protein is associated with a chloride ion channel. Examples of IBEM and the defective enzyme or protein are given in *Table 11.1*. Many hundreds of IBEMs have been described, most being extremely rare. It is the more common diseases that are more likely to be seen in the routine clinical biochemistry department. *Table 11.2* shows the incidence of some of the more well-known conditions.

Box 11.1 Biochemical genetics

Sir Archibald Garrod (1857–1936) was the founder of biochemical genetics. He studied the disease alcaptonuria, among others, at the beginning of the 20th century and showed that a chemical substance from the diet, which was not metabolized, appeared in the urine. His big deduction was that this was due to the absence of an enzyme, producing a metabolic block. It was not until 1958 that this was proved to be correct. His important work was ignored for 30 years before being recognized.

11.1   INHERITANCE

We inherit our genetic material through the chromosomes passed on from our mother and father: 23 pairs consisting of 22 pairs of autosomes and two sex chromosomes, which determine the sex of the individual. Inherited disease can be classified according to which type of chromosome the defective gene is found on (an autosome or a sex chromosome) and by the type of genetic expression shown by the gene. Each gene has two alleles (one from each parent), called the **genotype**. If these two alleles are identical, the individual is said to be **homozygous** for the characteristic expressed by the

Table 11.1 Some examples of inborn errors of metabolism and the affected enzyme/protein

Inborn error of metabolism	Affected enzyme/protein
Carbohydrate metabolism	
Glycogen storage disease	Various
Galactosaemia	Galactose-1-phosphate uridyl transferase
	Galactose kinase
Hereditary fructose intolerance	Fructose bisphosphate aldolase
Amino acid metabolism	
Phenylketonuria	Phenylalanine hydroxylase
Alkaptonuria	Homogentisic acid oxidase
Maple syrup urine disease	Branched-chain ketoacid dehydrogenase
Lipid metabolism	
Hyper- and hypolipoproteinaemia	Various
Steroid metabolism	
Congenital adrenal hyperplasia	21-Hydroxylase, 11β-hydroxylase
Purine metabolism	
Gout	Various
Lesch–Nyhan syndrome	Hypoxanthine-guanine phosphoribosyl transferase (HGPRT)
Lysosomal storage diseases	
Tay–Sachs disease	Hexosaminidase A
Gaucher's disease	Glycosylceramidase
Hurler's syndrome	Iduronidase
Cell transport defects	
Cystinuria	Amino acid transport
Renal glycosuria	Glucose transport
Renal tubular acidosis	Hydrogen ion transport
Cystic fibrosis	Chloride ion transport

Table 11.2. Approximate incidences of some inborn errors of metabolism in the Caucasian population

Cystic fibrosis	1:3000
Congenital hypothyroidism	1:4000
Phenylketonuria	1:10 000
Galactosaemia	1:50 000
Maple syrup urine disease	1:100 000

gene. This could be a normal enzyme or an inactive enzyme. If the two alleles are different, the individual is **heterozygous** for that characteristic. The inheritance patterns are different for autosomal and sex-linked genes. The probability of inheriting an abnormal gene for autosomal patterns of inheritance is shown in *Table 11.3*.

The expression of a characteristic depends on the dominance of the gene. A dominant gene will be expressed in both homozygous and heterozygous individuals with that gene. The characteristics of a recessive gene will only be expressed in a homozygous individual. In practice this is an oversimplification as many other factors can affect the expression of genes.

In sex-linked inheritance, expression depends on which chromosome the abnormal gene is found on. Males have one X and one Y chromosome and females have two X chromosomes. If the disease is X-linked, the abnormal gene is found on the X chromosome. Where a disease shows X-linked dominant characteristics, then both males and heterozygous females will be affected by gene expression. If the gene is a recessive gene, then it is males and only females homozygous for the abnormal gene who will be affected. Haemophilia is a well-known example of a disease inherited in this manner.

Table 11.3 Inheritance patterns for autosomal genes from homo- and heterozygous parents, showing the percentage chance of inheriting an abnormal gene (a) in a homozygous (Ho) or heterozygous (He) manner: the sum of the two numbers will give the total percentage chance of inheriting an abnormal gene*

Maternal genes	Paternal genes					
	A A		A a		a a	
	Ho	He	Ho	He	Ho	He
A A	0	0	0	50	0	100
A a	0	50	25	50	50	50
a a	0	100	50	50	100	0

*A = normal gene; a = abnormal gene.

11.2 INVESTIGATION OF IBEM

The investigation into an IBEM is an important role of the clinical biochemistry laboratory. Where the disease involves an enzyme defect there are four major biochemical changes that can be studied. These are:

- An accumulation of substrate before the enzyme defect;
- A decrease in the amount of product observed;
- An increased concentration of alternative metabolites;
- A decrease or absence of enzyme activity.

The essence of all biochemical investigation is based on these four observations (see *Fig. 11.1*), and the most commonly used is the demonstration of an increased amount of substrate or alternative metabolites. Definitive studies are required to demonstrate a lack of enzyme activity and these are usually performed on cells from the patient grown in cell culture. Modern molecular biology techniques are now used by specialist centres to detect the mutated gene. As examples of IBEM investigated by the clinical biochemistry laboratory, two well-known inherited diseases, phenylketonuria and cystic fibrosis, are discussed later in this chapter.

The investigation of IBEM can be divided into two distinct categories:

■ Screening for IBEM in individuals who do not have symptoms of a disease;
■ Investigation of patients with symptoms of IBEM.

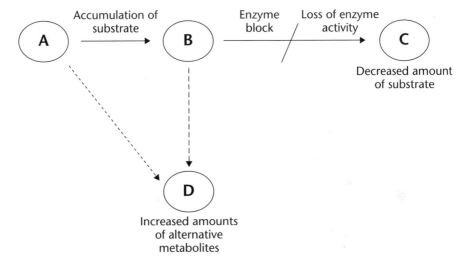

Figure 11.1
The four principal changes that can be observed in classical inborn errors of metabolism. The dashed arrows represent minor pathways.

Screening

Screening is the process of detecting a patient with an IBEM **before** they show overt symptoms of the disease. This allows suitable treatment to begin or relevant counselling to be given, depending on the situation. Screening for an IBEM is performed on patients who fall into one of a number of high-risk groups. These include:

■ All newborn infants;
■ Family of affected children;
■ Expectant mothers who have previously had affected children, i.e. **prenatal diagnosis**.

Screening all newborn infants is a great undertaking and will only be performed where the following conditions can be met:

■ There is a suitable treatment for the disease;
■ The disease is life-threatening or is seriously debilitating;
■ The disease has a relatively high incidence;
■ A suitable test is available;
■ The cost is acceptable.

Two diseases meet these criteria and national screening is now routinely performed on all newborn infants for phenylketonuria (PKU) and congenital hypothyroidism. Both conditions are easily treatable and have a simple test available. If left untreated, there are serious consequences for the patient and their family, with a considerable financial burden on health-care services.

The other screening tests are carried out on family members of an affected individual in order that carriers can be identified and appropriate genetic counselling given. This can help the parents decide if they will have further children. If they do decide to have further children then they may be offered prenatal screening for the disease.

Investigation of suspected IBEM

An IBEM may present with symptoms within the first few days or weeks of life. An infant may become very ill and display a number of symptoms that could suggest that they have an IBEM. These symptoms could be one or more of the following:

■ Failure to thrive;
■ Poor feeding;
■ Persistent vomiting;
■ Unexplained jaundice;
■ Unexplained hypoglycaemia;
■ Ketosis;
■ Lactic acidosis;
■ Convulsions and coma;
■ Lethargy;
■ Hypotonia;
■ Hyperventilation.

Other IBEMs present later, but usually within the first few years. In these cases, the patient may first display symptoms of abnormal liver function (see Chapter 18) or mental retardation.

In the biochemical investigation of these patients, a number of 'front-line' screening tests are performed, followed by a number of more specific tests. *Table 11.4* shows the more important tests used in the investigation of an IBEM.

Table 11.4 Biochemical tests performed in the investigation of a suspected inborn error of metabolism

Front-line tests	Follow-up tests	
Plasma	*Plasma:*	*Urine:*
Electrolytes	Insulin	Amino acids
Acid–base balance	Lactic acid	Organic acids
Blood gases	Ammonia	Sugars
Glucose	Ketones	
Liver function tests		
Calcium		

11.3 PRENATAL DIAGNOSIS

If parents with a previously affected child have further pregnancies they may be offered prenatal diagnosis to test if the foetus is affected. This can be performed on fibroblasts recovered from a sample of amniotic fluid taken by **amniocentesis**. The fibroblasts are cultured and specific enzyme studies are performed to check the activity of the enzyme that could be absent. Low activity or a lack of activity suggests that the foetus is affected.

Amniocentesis is carried out in the 15th week of pregnancy and the investigation should be complete by the 20th week. Another technique allows an earlier and more rapid diagnosis; this is **chorion villus biopsy**. In this technique, a sample of the chorion villus is taken at 9 weeks. DNA analysis for gene defects can be performed and the investigations completed within 10 days. This technique has been used to diagnose a number of inherited conditions such as cystic fibrosis.

More and more prenatal and other screening tests are being performed using newer molecular biology techniques to identify the abnormal gene and to make the diagnosis of the IBEM. In recent studies, methods of measuring specific foetal DNA in the maternal blood have shown the possibility of detecting inherited conditions in the foetus from a maternal blood sample. Chapter 4 gives an overview of the types of method used to analyse DNA.

11.4 PHENYLKETONURIA

Phenylketonuria (PKU) is an autosomal recessive disease with an incidence of approximately 1 in 10 000. It is caused by a deficiency in the enzyme phenylalanine hydroxylase, which converts phenylalanine into tyrosine (see *Fig. 11.2*). The consequence of the enzyme defect is that minor metabolic pathways become major routes for phenylalanine metabolism, leading to the excessive production of phenylketones – phenylpyruvate, phenylacetate and phenyllactate. These appear in the urine, hence the name of the condition.

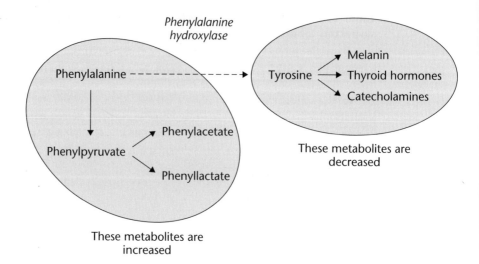

Figure 11.2
Biochemical changes seen in phenylketonuria due to the loss of activity of the enzyme phenylalanine hydroxylase.

In a small percentage of patients with PKU (3%), the defect is due to a deficiency in another enzyme which provides a cofactor necessary for the activation of phenylalanine hydroxylase (see *Box 11.2*).

Symptoms of the disease arise through lack of tyrosine and the toxic effects of phenylketones. The affected individual presents in the first few months of life with vomiting, irritability and seizures. They have fair hair, pale skin and blue eyes as a result of little melanin being produced. Mental retardation occurs from the age of 3–6 months. The ill-effects can be prevented or minimized if phenylalanine is excluded from the diet. Treatment of PKU involves placing the affected children on a special diet free from phenylalanine.

Box 11.2 Measuring phenylalanine

Phenylketones can be detected using the Guthrie test. This test uses a strain of *Bacillus subtilis* which will only grow in the presence of phenylalanine. Blood spots from patients with high levels of phenyl-alanine in their blood allow the bacteria to grow. Other laboratories measure phenylalanine chemically. If a cut-off of 240 µmol l^{-1} is used, 90% of positive results are due to causes other than PKU.

11.5 CYSTIC FIBROSIS

In addition to the classical IBEMs in which an enzyme is affected, it is now recognized that other proteins can be mutated, the inheritance of which can lead to a genetic disease that upsets the metabolic homeostasis of the cell and body. A good example of this type of IBEM is cystic fibrosis.

Cystic fibrosis is the most common genetic disease seen in the UK, with between 1 in 20 and 1 in 25 Caucasians being carriers of the disease. The cause of cystic fibrosis is a defective gene on chromosome 7 that codes for a protein called the cystic fibrosis transmembrane conductance regulator (CFTR). This protein normally regulates the passage of chloride ions across the cell membrane, and it is this regulatory function that is lost when a defective protein is produced as a result of inheriting the cystic fibrosis gene from both parents. The most common gene defect is the delta-F508 (ΔF508) mutation, accounting for about 70% of cases. This is the deletion of phenyl-alanine at position 508 in the CFTR protein.

Many organs are affected, particularly those which secrete fluids. In cystic fibrosis the normally watery fluids become thick and viscous like mucus and this allows bacteria to thrive and cause infections. The organs that are most commonly affected are the lungs, liver, pancreas, reproductive tract and skin. The lungs are gradually destroyed by repeated infections. The liver suffers damage from blockages in the bile ducts. Digestive enzymes are not delivered to the intestine from the pancreas, resulting in malnutrition. The reproductive tract may become blocked. In the skin, sweat glands produce an excess of salt in the perspiration.

The fact that the skin is unusually salty in patients with cystic fibrosis is the main feature by which the condition is currently diagnosed. Many laboratories measure the sodium and chloride in sweat; this is known as the **sweat test**. In this test sweat is collected on to preweighed filter paper discs. The weight of the sweat is determined by a second weighing following the collection of sweat. A known volume of water is added and the sodium and chloride are measured. A concentration greater than 45 mmol l^{-1} for sodium or chloride suggests cystic fibrosis. It is not unusual for affected children to have concentrations of around 100 mmol l^{-1}. In specialist centres there is a growing use of molecular biological techniques, for example PCR, for the screening and diagnosis of cystic fibrosis.

11.6 CHROMATOGRAPHY

In this chapter we shall examine one particular technique which has important applications in many fields of biochemistry, especially in the investigation of IBEM, and that is chromatography (see *Box 11.3*). This technique is important for separating complex mixtures of amino acids, organic acids, simple and complex sugars, and steroids, allowing the identification and

---

Box 11.3 Chromatography

Michel Tswett (1872–1919), a Russian botanist, was the inventor of chromatography. In 1933 he separated plant pigments by passing the mixture through a column of chalk powder.

measurement of an individual component in the sample. The investigation of an IBEM often relies on demonstrating a single component or a combination of particular components that are abnormally elevated as a result of a faulty enzyme. *Table 11.5* shows a number of analytes found in abnormally high amounts in various IBEMs.

Table 11.5 Examples of inborn errors of metabolism with the principal metabolites found in abnormally high concentrations

Metabolite	Inborn error of metabolism
Phenylalanine	Phenylketonuria
Homogentisic acid	Alkaptonuria
2-Oxoacids	Maple syrup urine disease
Galactose	Galactosaemia
Fructose-1-phosphate	Hereditary fructose intolerance
Uric acid	Lesch–Nyhan syndrome
11-Deoxycortisol and 11-deoxycorticosterone	Congenital adrenal hyperplasia

Literally meaning 'colour writing', chromatography is the term used to describe a technique that can separate a mixture of compounds into individual components, which can then be identified and quantified. Essentially, chromatography involves a **mobile phase**, containing the dissolved sample, flowing across a **stationary phase**. Separation of the dissolved components in the sample occurs as a result of components being retarded by differing extents by the stationary phase. There are many forms of chromatography, using a wide range of mobile and stationary phases and methods of detecting the presence of separated compounds. The simplest technique is thin-layer chromatography (TLC), the theory of which can serve as a model for other types of chromatography. TLC uses only a few microlitres of sample, which are dried on to a thin layer of silica gel that has been spread thinly over a plastic or glass support, called a **plate**. The plate is placed vertically in a few millimetres of solvent, often a mixture of methanol and water, which flows up the plate by capillary action. As the solvent flows up the plate the sample is carried with it and components within the sample are separated, depending on the relative physical attraction between them and the silica solid phase. Those components that show no interaction (or attraction) with the silica stationary phase will be carried at the solvent front. Components, or molecules, that show interaction with the silica stationary phase are retarded and travel more slowly. The greater the interaction between a molecule in the sample and the solid phase, the slower it will travel up the plate. Separated compounds are visualized using a developing solution, which reacts with the compound on the silica to produce a coloured compound that can be seen by eye. The distance travelled by a compound is measured and compared with the distance travelled by the solvent front. By dividing one distance by the other, the **Rf** ('relative to the front') value for that compound is found. The Rf value for a given compound, separated under identical conditions, will always be constant, aiding in the identification of the separated compound.

$$Rf = \frac{\text{Distance travelled by the compound}}{\text{Distance travelled by solvent front}}$$

A sample that is not retarded by the silica solid phase will move with the solvent front and will have an Rf value of 1.0, whereas a compound that travels half the distance (compared with the solvent) will have an Rf value of 0.5.

This principle, where different molecules in the sample interact with the solid phase to differing extents and are thereby separated, holds true for all types of chromatography. *Table 11.6* lists the major types of chromatography found in the clinical biochemistry laboratory together with an example of an application.

Table 11.6 Examples of applications for types of chromatographic technique

Technique	Application
Thin-layer chromatography (TLC)	Rapid screening for urinary sugars
High-performance liquid chromatography (HPLC)	Analysis of some fatty acids and small molecules
Gas–liquid chromatography (GLC)	Measuring levels of steroids and volatile organic compounds

TLC is a particularly useful technique for screening many samples for drugs of abuse. Using different developing solutions, many different drugs can be identified. High-performance liquid chromatography (HPLC) and gas–liquid chromatography (GLC) are specialized techniques using sophisticated instrumentation. HPLC is useful for the separation and identification of many biological substances, usually small molecules. GLC complements HPLC, being used for the separation of volatile organic compounds. Derivatives of compounds can be made, making them volatile, and thereby enabling them to be measured by GLC. Many drugs can also be measured by GLC.

SUGGESTED FURTHER READING

In addition to relevant chapters in the text books cited in Chapter 1 the following references are recommended.

Bamforth F.J. (1994) Laboratory screening for genetic disorders and birth defects. *Clinical Biochemistry*, **27**: 333–342.

Fernandes J., Saudubray J.-M., van den Berghe G. and Walter J.H. (eds) (2006) *Inborn Metabolic Diseases: Diagnosis and Treatment*, 4th edition. Heidelberg: Springer-Verlag.

Nyhan W.L. and Barshop B.A. (2005) *Atlas of Metabolic Diseases*, 2nd edition. London: Hodder Arnold.

Rashed M.S. (2001) Clinical applications of tandem mass spectrometry: ten years of diagnosis and screening for inherited metabolic diseases. *Journal of Chromatography B: Biomedical Sciences and Applications*, **758**: 27–48.

Velázquez A., Vela-Amieva M., Cicerón-Arellano I., *et al.* (2000) Diagnosis of inborn errors of metabolism. *Archives of Medical Research*, **31**: 145–150.

SELF-ASSESSMENT QUESTIONS

1. What is the most common enzyme defect in PKU?
2. What is the probability of inheriting an affected autosomal gene from two carrier parents?
3. What is the probability of a child of two carrier parents expressing an autosomal recessive disease?
4. What is screening designed to do?
5. Which three types of compound are looked for in urine samples in the laboratory investigation of an inborn error of metabolism?
6. How are fibroblasts obtained for prenatal diagnosis?
7. In cystic fibrosis, what is the most common mutation?
8. Name a chromatographic technique suitable for the rapid screening of urinary sugars.
9. What is the major metabolite that accumulates in alkaptonuria?
10. Which three metabolic changes are seen in a classical inborn error of metabolism where there is an enzyme defect?

Plasma proteins

> **Learning objectives**
> *After studying this chapter you should confidently be able to:*
>
> ■ **Describe the roles of plasma proteins.**
> Total protein is composed of albumin and globulins. The roles of different proteins include transport, storage, defence and maintaining the osmotic pressure.
>
> ■ **Describe the role of important specific proteins.**
> Albumin is synthesized in the liver and is important for maintaining oncotic pressure. Caeruloplasmin is a copper-containing protein that is elevated in Wilson's disease. Transferrin is an iron-containing protein useful in the investigation of anaemia. α_1-Foetoprotein is useful in the detection of neural tube defects and Down syndrome. Prostate-specific antigen is elevated in prostate cancer. C-reactive protein is elevated in cases of inflammation and infection. Tumour markers can be used to detect cancer and monitor cancer therapy.
>
> ■ **Explain protein separation by electrophoresis.**
> Plasma proteins can be separated into a number of discrete bands by electrophoresis. The pH at which a protein has a zero net charge is the isoelectric point. Most proteins are negatively charged and migrate towards the positive electrode (anode) in electrophoresis.

In this section we shall be looking at aspects of **transport and storage** in the body. In particular we shall study the areas where disease processes cause biochemical changes detectable in the blood, which can be investigated in the clinical biochemistry laboratory. Transport of materials such as products of digestion or waste products is important to maintain the smooth running and health of the body. Proteins are important transport molecules and are discussed in this chapter. Proteins are also important in the transport of lipids and a more detailed study of their role in lipid metabolism is given in the next chapter. Gas transport is vital for life and is involved in the removal and normal regulation of hydrogen ions, and this is considered in more detail in Chapter 14.

The proteins being considered in this chapter are the plasma proteins, most of which are synthesized within the liver. Although this chapter is in the section primarily dealing with transport, the plasma proteins have a wider range of functions:

- Transport;
- Storage;
- Defence (this is considered in the next section);
- Blood clotting;
- Maintenance of osmotic pressure (discussed in Chapter 7).

In blood, the plasma proteins have an important role in the transport of a number of different components. As we shall see in Chapter 14, an important protein found within red blood cells is essential for transporting oxygen; this protein is haemoglobin. *Table 12.1* lists some of the major transport proteins found in plasma (see *Box 12.1*).

Table 12.1 Examples of transport proteins found in plasma

Plasma protein	Transported molecule
Pre-albumin	Vitamin A, thyroid hormones
Albumin	Calcium, thyroid hormones, drugs, bilirubin, amino acids
Transferrin	Iron
Caeruloplasmin	Copper
Hormone-binding proteins	Thyroid hormones, sex hormones, cortisol, e.g. cortisol-binding protein
Lipoproteins	Lipids

Box 12.1 Proteins

The word 'protein' is derived from the Greek word *proteios,* meaning 'first.' It was introduced by the Dutch chemist Mulder in the late 1830s and implied that proteins were substances of primary importance in the body.

The investigation of plasma proteins in disease by the clinical laboratory can be considered in two ways: the first is the measurement of total protein and the relative distribution of the major proteins, and the second is the measurement of specific proteins in the plasma. The first approach is not specific for any one pathological condition but can act as a screening test for many different conditions. The second approach, where a specific protein is measured (apart from albumin), can give information about particular diseases (see *Box 12.2*).

Box 12.2 Protein shape and structure

The three-dimensional shape of proteins allows the wide range of functions we observe. The charge associated with particular amino acids at particular points on the surface of the protein molecule allows it to bind specifically to many thousands of other proteins and smaller molecules. The shape of proteins can be determined using sophisticated techniques such as X-ray crystallography. Dorothy Hodgkin was one of the first scientists to use this technique to deduce the structure of complex molecules. In 1972 she was able to describe the detailed structure of insulin, a protein with over 800 atoms.

12.1 TOTAL PROTEIN

Total protein measurement is a fairly non-specific measurement as it can be influenced by many variables, and thus changes in one protein or group of proteins can be masked by opposite changes in other proteins. For example, a decreased concentration of one protein is masked by an increased concentration of another. Total protein measurements can give an indication of gross changes brought about by a number of different disease states (see *Box 12.3*). An increased concentration of total protein can be due to:

■ An increase in an individual protein or group of proteins;
■ An increase in all proteins.

A common example of an individual protein causing an elevated total protein result is in conditions that cause high levels of antibodies to be produced. More commonly, an elevated total protein level is caused by dehydration of the patient, where fluid has been lost and therefore the same amount of dissolved protein is present in a smaller volume of fluid, resulting in a higher concentration. Any condition that results in dehydration will show an increased total protein concentration in the blood. Sometimes the elevated total protein level is an artefact due to excessive stasis when the blood sample was taken. Stasis results from too much pressure being applied to the arm, which makes the vein more accessible but causes fluid to be forced from the blood vessel into the surrounding tissue, thereby causing a localized increase in the protein concentration.

Low total protein levels in the blood can be found in cases of severe disease such as liver disease or severe malnutrition where the synthesis of protein is reduced. More commonly, low total protein levels are found in situations where there is dilution of the blood (haemodilution) caused by

---

Box 12.3 Amino acid sequences of proteins

Frederick Sanger developed a method for determining the amino acid sequence of proteins in the early 1940s. He was awarded two Nobel Prizes (in 1958 and 1980) for his work on determining the structure of proteins and nucleic acids.

overhydration. Total protein levels can also be affected by the absence of one of the major blood proteins, for example, hypoalbuminaemia or hypogammaglobulinaemia.

12.2 PROTEIN GROUPS

Total protein measurements do not by themselves often provide useful clinical information. Of more importance is the overall pattern of proteins present in the blood. To obtain this information the total proteins are separated into a number of distinct groups, and this is achieved using electrophoresis (described later in the chapter). Proteins are separated by their charge. *Figure 12.1* shows an **electrophoretic separation** of serum proteins. The major band is **albumin** and the remaining five bands are called the **globulins**. The globulin concentration is easily found by subtracting the albumin concentration from the total protein concentration. Electrophoresis separates the globulins into five bands, which are a mixture of proteins that migrate together in the electric field. The name and composition of the globulin bands is given in *Table 12.2*.

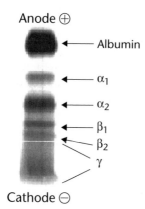

Anode ⊕

Albumin

α_1

α_2

β_1

β_2

γ

Cathode ⊖

Figure 12.1
The major bands identified on an electrophoresis strip. See *Table 12.2* for details of the most important proteins that migrate to each region.

If special high-resolution techniques are used, the proteins may separate into 15–20 separate bands. The electrophoretic pattern can be inspected visually to give much information about the patient. Electrophoresis gives information about many different conditions, as the intensity of the different protein bands varies in different diseases. Protein changes, and therefore changes in the electrophoretic pattern, are seen in liver disease, kidney disease, inflammatory conditions, infections, some cancers and in conditions that affect a specific protein.

Table 12.2 The major proteins found in the globulin bands after separation by agarose electrophoresis

Electrophoresis band	Major proteins
α_1-Globulins	α_1-Antitrypsin α_1-Acid glycoprotein (orosomucoid) α-Lipoprotein
α_2-Globulins	Haptoglobin Caeruloplasmin α_2-Macroglobulin
β_1-Globulins	Transferrin β-Lipoprotein
β_2-Globulins	C3 Fibrinogen (only in plasma)
γ-Globulins	Immunoglobulins

12.3 SPECIFIC PROTEINS

A number of specific proteins are important in the diagnosis of certain conditions, whilst some of the measurements are not specific to any particular disease but give a more general picture of the state of health for a given patient, for example albumin. Other protein measurements give information concerning a particular disease; for example, caeruloplasmin is important in the diagnosis of Wilson's disease, a disease of copper metabolism. Some of the clinically important proteins measured in the clinical biochemistry laboratory are given below.

Albumin (molecular weight 66 kDa)

Albumin is the most abundant protein found in the plasma, making up 55–65% of the total protein (reference range 35–50 g l^{-1}). Albumin is synthesized by the liver and is the most important protein in maintaining the oncotic pressure of plasma. Another important role of this protein is that of a non-specific transport protein, as it binds many non-polar compounds such as bilirubin, long-chain fatty acids and a number of drugs. Albumin also functions as a reservoir for a number of hormones, particularly thyroid hormones.

Abnormal levels of albumin are not diagnostic of any particular disease. High levels (**hyperalbuminaemia**) are only found in dehydrated patients and are of little diagnostic value. Low albumin levels (**hypoalbuminaemia**) are found in many conditions where there is:

- Impaired synthesis as a result of liver disease;
- Increased breakdown of protein due to tissue damage or inflammation;

■ Reduced absorption of amino acids, as seen in conditions leading to malabsorption or in cases of malnutrition;

■ Increased protein loss associated with renal disease, protein-losing enteropathy or severe burns.

Very low albumin levels, below 25 g l^{-1}, result in a loss of plasma oncotic pressure and cause movement of fluid from the circulatory system into the tissue, causing oedema. The low levels also act to modify the ratio of bound to free levels of substances that bind to albumin; this can affect levels of hormones and calcium concentration in the blood in particular.

Caeruloplasmin (molecular weight 132 kDa)

Caeruloplasmin is the major copper-containing protein found in plasma. It contains between six and seven copper atoms per molecule. It has a plasma concentration of approximately 0.35 g l^{-1}. It was thought that caeruloplasmin was a copper transport protein, but more recent evidence would suggest that the major role for caeruloplasmin is as an antioxidant. Caeruloplasmin has an important role to play in the diagnosis of **Wilson's disease**. This is a rare defect of copper metabolism where deposition of copper occurs in the liver, kidneys and brain. Copper is also deposited in the cornea, giving rise to characteristic rings called **Kayser–Fleischer** rings. Low levels of caeruloplasmin are found in this condition but may also be found in patients with malnutrition, malabsorption, severe liver disease and nephrotic syndrome.

Transferrin (molecular weight 78 kDa)

Transferrin is the major plasma protein transporting iron (reference range 2.2–4.0 g l^{-1}). The liver is the major organ for transferrin synthesis, which appears to be controlled by the iron concentration in the blood. Low iron levels result in more transferrin being synthesized and, as the iron levels increase, the transferrin levels return to normal. The measurement of transferrin is of most use in the differential diagnosis of anaemia. Common iron deficiency will result in an increase in transferrin.

α_1-Foetoprotein (molecular weight 69 kDa)

α_1-Foetoprotein is the major foetal plasma protein and rapidly disappears after birth. It has a similar role to albumin but it may also be involved in the immunoregulation of pregnancy. In the clinical laboratory α_1-foetoprotein measurement has important diagnostic applications. The first is in the prenatal diagnosis of neural tube defects in the developing foetus and, more recently, of Down syndrome. High levels of α_1-foetoprotein are found in the amniotic fluid and maternal plasma from women carrying a foetus with an open neural tube defect. Down syndrome is associated with low concentrations of α_1-foetoprotein in the mother's blood and the level is often used in conjunction with other measurements, namely β human chorionic gonadotrophin and estradiol, to calculate a risk assessment of that mother having a baby affected with Down syndrome. Screening programmes are widely used to screen all pregnant women, if they wish, for neural tube defects and Down syndrome, with the clinical biochemistry laboratory playing an important role.

The second diagnostic application of α_1-foetoprotein is in the detection of liver cancer. In approximately 80% of adults with liver cancer, there is a marked rise in α_1-foetoprotein concentration – normally only a trace of α_1-foetoprotein can be detected in adult blood (less than 15 µg l^{-1}). Measurement of sequential blood levels is particularly useful for monitoring therapy and assessing the prognosis of the patient.

Prostate-specific antigen (molecular weight 33 kDa)

Prostate-specific antigen (PSA) is an enzyme (a serine protease) normally found only in the prostate gland. Only very low levels are normally detected in plasma (reference range <4.0 µg l^{-1}). Levels higher than this can indicate cancer of the prostate but can also indicate benign prostatic hypertrophy. The higher the PSA level in the blood, the greater the chance of that patient having prostate cancer. Levels into the thousands of micrograms have been known with patients suffering advanced cancer. The monitoring of blood PSA levels every 6 months can be useful in monitoring the effectiveness of treatment and control of the disease.

C-reactive protein (molecular weight 105 kDa)

C-reactive protein (CRP) is synthesized in the liver and is made up of five identical subunits. This protein is a member of a group of proteins called the acute-phase proteins (which are discussed in more detail in Chapter 16). CRP is important in protecting the body from bacterial infection and is involved in activating complement. Elevated levels are seen in a wide range of conditions that result in inflammation, for example in infections and other inflammatory diseases such as rheumatoid arthritis. CRP is a non-specific marker for inflammation and can show a massive increase in plasma concentrations. The plasma concentration is normally less than 8 mg l^{-1}, but infection may increase this concentration by at least a hundredfold.

Immunoglobulin (molecular weight 150–900 kDa)

Immunoglobulins are antibodies and are important in the prevention of infection. There are five classes of immunoglobin, which are discussed in detail in Chapter 15 along with their clinical significance.

Enzymes

Many clinically important proteins are enzymes and these are measured using their intrinsic enzymatic activity. Chapter 10 discusses the clinically important plasma enzymes in detail.

Tumour markers

Many proteins measured in the clinical biochemistry laboratory are useful in the diagnosis and monitoring of cancer. Different biochemical markers can be associated with particular cancers; for example, PSA is a marker of prostate cancer. Many tumours modify the levels of proteins normally found in the plasma and these are usually enzymes. Other tumour markers are synthesized by the tumour itself and may be a foetal protein, not normally expressed by adult cells. A good example of this is the tumour marker associated with colorectal cancer: carcinoembryonic antigen. A number of glycoproteins have been identified with specific tumours; these are called carbohydrate antigens (CA) and can be detected on the surface of tumour cells and also measured in blood samples. It must be remembered that many abnormal hormone levels may be due to a tumour of endocrine tissue. *Table 12.3* gives examples of common biochemical tumour markers that are measured in the laboratory and the major cancers associated with them.

Table 12.3 Commonly measured biochemical tumour markers and the associated tissue of tumour origin

Tumour marker	Cancer
Enzymes	
Acid phosphatase	Prostate
Alkaline phosphatase	Bone, liver
Prostate-specific antigen	Prostate
Proteins	
Carcinoembryonic antigen	Colon, bronchus
α_1-Foetoprotein	Liver
Immunoglobulins	Plasma cells
Carbohydrate antigens	
CA 125	Ovary
CA 15-3	Breast

12.4 MEASUREMENT OF PLASMA PROTEINS

The investigation of proteins in plasma samples falls into two categories, the first being the measure of total protein and the second being the measurement of an individual protein. There are many different methods available for measuring proteins and the method chosen will depend on whether an individual protein, a group of proteins or total protein is to be measured. *Table 12.4* gives a selection of methods used to measure proteins in the clinical biochemistry laboratory.

Table 12.4 Commonly used techniques for measuring proteins in biological fluids

Method	Use
Chemical reactions producing a coloured product	Total protein
Ultraviolet absorption at 200–225 nm and 270–290 nm	Total protein
Precipitation methods	Total protein
Dye-binding methods	Total protein, albumin
Refractometry	Total protein
Electrophoretic methods	Total and specific proteins
Immunoassay	Specific proteins

Total protein

A number of different methods are available for measuring total proteins. Most commonly the method used is a chemical reaction to produce a colour; for example, the **Biuret** method, which measures the colour formed when copper ions react with the peptide bonds found in all proteins. The advantage of the chemical reaction is that it can very easily be automated, allowing large numbers of samples to be measured rapidly. **Refractometry** is a very simple method where the refractive index of the sample is measured, this being a direct measurement of the total protein concentration. This is a simple and rapid technique and can be used where there are only a few samples to be analysed.

Total protein measurement is non-specific, giving limited information, and in some situations it is necessary to measure an individual protein to aid in the diagnosis of a particular disease. In order to do this it is necessary to separate that protein from the other proteins in the sample or to use a method that is highly specific for that protein.

Electrophoresis

Electrophoresis is a technique commonly used to separate the serum proteins into a number of bands called an **electrophoretogram** or **electrophoresis strip**, using an electric current. The electrophoresis strip is inspected visually and can be used to screen for a number of diseases (see *Box 12.4*).

Electrophoresis is the movement of charged particles in an electric field.

Box 12.4 Electrophoresis

Electrophoresis was discovered by the Swedish biochemist Arne Tiselius (1902–1971) in Uppsala, Sweden. He showed that blood proteins in serum could be separated into four major bands by applying an electric current. He was awarded a Nobel Prize in 1948 for his work in this area.

Proteins have a net charge derived from the ionization of amino acid residues that make up the protein. The exact charge on the protein molecule will depend on the pH of the solution in which the protein is dissolved. At high pH values, where there is a lack of hydrogen ions, the protein will be negatively charged. Conversely, at low pH values where there is an abundance of hydrogen ions, the protein will have a positive charge. At a particular pH the protein molecule will have an equivalent number of positive and negative charges resulting in a net charge of zero. The pH at which the protein has a net charge of zero is called the **isoelectric point** (pI).

A diagram of an electrophoresis apparatus is shown in *Fig. 12.2*. Here, the sample is placed in a buffer, usually at pH 8.6, which gives most of the proteins in the sample a negative charge. The sample is allowed to soak into a gel such as agarose. In most cases the amount of sample loaded is only a few microlitres. A voltage is applied and current passes through the gel via electrode wicks dipped in electrophoresis buffer and placed in contact with the gel surface. Usually a voltage of 100–200 V is applied. Proteins migrate through the agarose gel and form the bands seen in *Fig. 12.1*. Proteins with a large negative charge will move more rapidly towards the positive electrode (**anode**) than those with a smaller negative charge. Some proteins will have a positive charge and will move towards the negative electrode (**cathode**), and the greater the positive charge, the quicker the migration of the protein. Typically, an electrophoresis run will take from 30 minutes up to an hour for separation of the bands to occur. A more recent development called

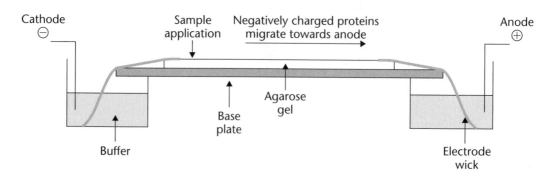

Figure 12.2

Electrophoresis apparatus used in the separation of proteins in a sample loaded on to an agarose gel.

capillary electrophoresis allows proteins to be separated and quantitated in only a few minutes, using voltages as high as 30 000 V!

When the separation is finished the protein bands are stained with a protein stain, allowing the separated bands to be seen. Coomassie Brilliant Blue is commonly used for this, although other stains can be used such as Ponceau Red.

Electrophoresis is a powerful technique for screening serum samples for a number of diseases, in particular the detection of an abnormal antibody pattern, as discussed in more detail in Chapter 15. The electrophoretic pattern can be assessed by eye to give a qualitative assessment of the protein pattern or the electrophoretic strip can be scanned in a scanning densitometer to give a semi-quantitative measurement of a protein band.

Other electrophoretic techniques allow separation of proteins according to their molecular weight or their isoelectric point. A powerful combination of these two electrophoretic methods is now being widely used to discover new proteins expressed in diseases such as cancer. This technique, called two-dimensional electrophoresis, separates proteins by their molecular weight in one direction and by their isoelectric point in a second direction, giving rise to a two-dimensional pattern of many hundreds of protein spots. Careful analysis of the data can reveal proteins expressed by diseased cells. *Figure 12.3* shows an example of a two-dimensional electrophoresis separation. These techniques are usually restricted to more specialized laboratories or research laboratories and are not often used in the routine clinical laboratory.

The measurement of specific proteins is nowadays performed using an immunoassay, where the antibody used specifically reacts with the protein of interest. These immunoassays can be easily automated and many samples

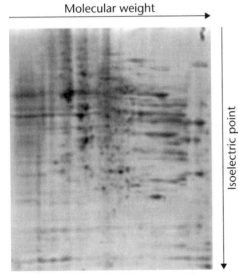

Figure 12.3
Section from a two-dimensional separation of proteins. The proteins are separated by their molecular weight in one dimension and by their isoelectric point in the other.

analysed quickly on large laboratory analysers. Immunoassays are discussed in greater detail in Chapters 5 and 6.

SUGGESTED FURTHER READING

In addition to relevant chapters in the text books cited in Chapter 1 the following references are recommended.

Bossuyt X. (2006) Advances in serum protein electrophoresis. *Advances in Clinical Chemistry*, **42**: 43–80.

Duffy M.J. (2007) Role of tumor markers in patients with solid cancers: a critical review. *European Journal of Internal Medicine*, **18**: 175–184.

Gion M. (2000) Serum tumour markers: from quality control to total quality management. *The Breast*, **9**: 306–311.

Keren D.F. (2003) *Protein Electrophoresis in Clinical Diagnosis*. London: Hodder Arnold.

Roddam A.W., Duffy M.J., Hamdy F.C., *et al.* (2005) The use of prostate-specific antigen (PSA) isoforms for the detection of prostate cancer in men with a PSA level of 2–10 ng/ml: systematic review and meta-analysis. NHS Prostate Cancer Risk Management Programme. *European Urology*, **48**: 386–399.

Schaller J., Gerber S., Kaempfer U., Trachsel C. and Lejon S. (2007) *Human Blood Plasma Proteins*. New York: John Wiley & Sons Ltd.

SELF-ASSESSMENT QUESTIONS

1. Which protein is found transporting iron in plasma?
2. Where are most plasma proteins synthesized?
3. What is the most abundant protein present in plasma?
4. What are the major proteins found in the α_2 globulin band?
5. Below what concentration of plasma albumin will there be a reduction in the plasma oncotic pressure?
6. Which protein can be used as a tumour marker for prostate cancer?
7. Immunoassays are useful for measuring the concentration of what types of protein?
8. What is the name given to the pH at which a protein molecule has a net charge of zero?
9. At pH 8.6, which electrode will most plasma proteins migrate towards?

Lipids and lipoproteins

Learning objectives
After studying this chapter you should confidently be able to:

■ **Describe different types of lipid and lipoprotein.**
There are four major forms of lipid: cholesterol, triglyceride, phospholipid and fatty acids. Lipids are transported in packages called lipoproteins, which are composed of cholesterol, triglyceride, phospholipid and apolipoprotein. The important lipoproteins are chylomicrons, VLDL, IDL, LDL and HDL, where each lipoprotein represents a different stage in the transport of lipid.

■ **Review different types of lipid disorder.**
The primary hyperlipidaemias are classified by the WHO into six categories. The WHO, or Fredrickson, classification is based on plasma analysis. Hypolipidaemias are rare and are usually associated with an apolipoprotein deficiency.

■ **Describe the types of lipid disorder.**
The majority of hyperlipidaemias are classified as primary (the most common), familial conditions and secondary hyperlipidaemia. Hypolidipaemia is rare. Atherosclerosis is a common disease associated with lipids and lipoproteins. Increased levels of LDL and lipoprotein-(a) correlate with an increased risk of heart disease. Increased levels of HDL and lipoprotein-(a) correlate with a decreased risk of heart disease.

■ **Give an overview of the methodology used to measure plasma lipids.**
Investigations of lipids should be performed on a fasting blood sample. Measurement of cholesterol and triglyceride is based on an enzyme assay generating a product in proportion to the blood concentration of cholesterol or trigyceride. Investigation into lipoproteins is by electrophoresis or immunoassay.

In this chapter we will consider the transport of lipid and diseases associated with impaired lipid handling. As we saw in Chapter 2, lipid is an important source and store of energy. Lipid is a name given to compounds which are insoluble in water, and this property requires that lipid be transported bound to other molecules, to enable it to be transported in an aqueous environment. There are four major groups of lipid: **cholesterol**, **triglyceride**, **phospholipid** and **fatty acids**. Cholesterol is present in the diet and is required by all cells (see *Box 13.1*). Cells can synthesize cholesterol, which is the precursor for the steroid hormones and is mostly made in the adrenal glands and the gonads. Triglyceride is the major lipid found in the diet and is broken down to yield glycerol and fatty acids. Related to triglyceride is phospholipid, which has a similar structure to triglyceride but with one of the fatty acids being replaced by a polar group. This gives phospholipid an important detergent-like property, having both polar and non-polar groups within the same molecule. Lastly, there are fatty acids, which are usually straight-chain monocarboxylic acids derived from triglyceride. The body can synthesize most fatty acids but there are some that cannot be synthesized, the so-called essential fatty acids (see Chapter 2).

Box 13.1 Cholesterol

Cholesterol is an alicyclic sterol, $C_{27}H_{45}OH$, with molecular weight 386. It is a white crystalline solid with a melting point of 148.5°C. It is the parent compound for all the steroid hormones.

13.1 LIPIDS AND LIPOPROTEINS

Lipid is transported in the blood in small particles called lipoproteins, which are synthesized in the liver and gut. These particles are a complex of triglyceride, cholesterol, phospholipid and proteins. The lipoprotein particles range in size from 10 to 500 nm and have a hydrophobic core and a hydrophilic outer shell. Phospholipid and cholesterol have both hydrophobic and hydrophilic 'ends' of the molecule; the hydrophilic ends face outwards and the hydrophobic ends make up the core with triglyceride. These bipolar lipids form a micelle in which the proteins are embedded. *Figure 13.1* shows this arrangement. The proteins associated with the

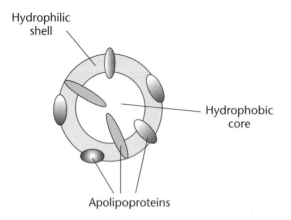

Figure 13.1
A lipoprotein, showing the hydrophobic core, hydrophilic shell and embedded apolipoproteins.

lipoprotein are called **apolipoproteins** and they perform a number of functions such as activating enzymes and regulating the binding of lipoprotein to cell surface receptors. *Table 13.1* lists the major apolipoproteins together with their function.

There are five main types of lipoprotein, classified according to size and density. Each type has a different composition of lipid and a different number of apolipoproteins in the complex. The five lipoproteins, in decreasing order of size are: chylomicrons, very-low-density lipoprotein (VLDL), intermediate-density lipoprotein (IDL), low-density lipoprotein (LDL) and high-density lipoprotein (HDL). *Table 13.2* shows the physical properties and composition of these lipoproteins.

Table 13.1 The major groups of apolipoprotein and their functions

Apolipoprotein	Function
Apo A	Enzyme cofactors
Apo B	Receptor binding
Apo C	Enzyme cofactors and inhibitors
Apo E	Receptor binding

Table 13.2 Properties of lipoproteins

	Chylomicrons	VLDL	IDL	LDL	HDL
Diameter (nm)	100–500	30–80	25–30	18–30	5–12
Approximate density (g ml^{-1})	0.94	1.002	1.012	1.04	>1.06
% Triglyceride	90	65	35	10	5
% Cholesterol	4.5	20	40	50	35
% Phospholipid	4.5	10	15	20	35
% Protein	1	5	10	20	25
Major apolipoprotein composition	B, C, E	C, B, E	B	B	A, C, E

Chylomicrons

Chylomicrons are the largest particles and are rich in triglyceride. Their main function is to transport lipid from the gut, via the lymphatic and circulatory systems, to adipose and muscle cells. As triglyceride is removed from the chylomicron, the particle becomes smaller and of a higher cholesterol composition. The remnant chylomicrons are removed from the circulation by the liver.

Very-low-density lipoprotein

These medium-sized particles, containing mainly triglyceride, are synthesized in the liver. The main function of VLDL is to transport lipids synthesized in the liver to parts of the body that require triglyceride as an energy source or for storage.

Intermediate-density lipoprotein

These lipoproteins are derived from VLDL particles and are an intermediate in the conversion of VLDL to LDL.

Low-density lipoprotein

These are small particles rich in cholesterol derived from the metabolism of VLDL. They contain an important apolipoprotein called apo B-100, which is responsible for recognizing an LDL receptor on the surface of cells.

High-density lipoprotein

HDL is the smallest of the lipoproteins, but the most dense, and contains the highest protein concentration. The role of HDL is to remove cholesterol from peripheral cells and plasma, transporting the cholesterol to the liver for reprocessing or excretion.

13.2   LIPID TRANSPORT

Exogenous lipid

Figure 13.2 shows an overview of lipid transport as described in more detail below. Dietary lipids are digested and absorbed in the gut through the intestinal mucosal cells. The products of lipid digestion, namely free fatty acids and triglycerides, are esterified. Cholesterol is also absorbed and some is esterified. The lipids are assembled with a number of proteins, called apolipoproteins, into a package called a chylomicron. Chylomicrons travel through the lymphatic system and enter the blood stream. The chylomicrons are rich in triglyceride and cholesterol. In the circulation an enzyme called lipoprotein lipase acts on chylomicrons to release fatty acids and glycerol. Lipoprotein lipase is found on the surface of the endothelial cells lining blood capillaries, especially in adipose and muscle tissue. Adipose cells absorb the fatty acids and glycerol to synthesize triglyceride, which is stored

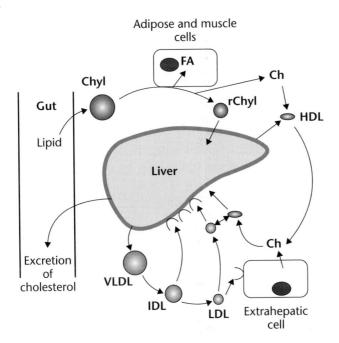

Figure 13.2
An overview of lipoprotein metabolism. Chyl = chylomicron; rChyl = remnant chylomicron; VLDL = very-low-density lipoprotein; IDL = intermediate-density lipoprotein; LDL = low-density lipoprotein; HDL = high-density lipoprotein; FA = fatty acid; Ch = cholesterol.

within the cell as fat, whilst muscle cells use the released lipids as a source of energy. The liver uses released glycerol to synthesize more triglyceride and phospholipid. The chylomicron becomes smaller as lipid is digested and released, forming a remnant chylomicron, which is rapidly removed by the liver.

Endogenous lipid

Lipid is synthesized within the liver and is transported via the blood to extrahepatic cells where the lipid is used by the cell in its metabolism. In the hepatocytes, cholesterol and triglyceride are assembled into a package with a number of apolipoproteins. This large package is rich in lipid and has a very low density and so is referred to as VLDL. VLDL is released into the circulation and initially its metabolism is similar to that of chylomicrons. Lipoprotein lipase releases fatty acids and glycerol which are taken up by cells and, as a result, the lipid content drops and the particles become more dense, forming IDL. In doing so, the particle loses some of its protein content. Some IDL is taken up by the liver but most loses more triglyceride and becomes LDL. LDL is smaller and denser than IDL; it is also rich in cholesterol and is the main carrier of cholesterol in the blood. Receptors on the surface of cells, called LDL receptors, recognize the remaining apolipoprotein, apo B-100, in the LDL particle and cause the LDL to bind to the cell surface and be taken into the cell, where cholesterol is released. Nearly all LDL is removed from the blood by this receptor-mediated pathway. Any receptor defect can lead to an inefficient uptake and clearance of LDL. Uptake of LDL by receptors is regulated by the cell's requirement for cholesterol and, as such, it is a regulated pathway. There is also an unregulated pathway which operates when the blood cholesterol level is high, whereby cholesterol is taken up directly by cells, particularly macrophages. The liver has the highest concentration of LDL receptors in the body and other tissues that require high amounts of cholesterol have high levels of LDL receptors on the surface of their cells. In particular, the adrenal cortex and the gonads bind LDL and the cholesterol is used in the synthesis of steroid hormones.

The degradation of chylomicrons releases cholesterol into the plasma and cells can release cholesterol into the plasma. The liver synthesizes HDL particles that remove free cholesterol from the plasma and esterify it to produce cholesterol esters. The HDL transports cholesterol back to the liver where it is taken up by the hepatocytes and excreted in the bile. Another part of this mechanism involves the transfer of cholesterol ester to LDL in exchange for cholesterol, which is also esterified by the HDL.

13.3 LIPID DISORDERS

In the investigation of lipid disorders it is the presence of high lipid levels (**hyperlipidaemia**) that is important. Hyperlipidaemia can be either a primary disorder or secondary to another pathological process. Primary causes of hyperlipidaemia arise from gene defects of lipoprotein or lipoprotein receptors. Often there is a combination of genetic and environmental factors leading to hyperlipidaemia.

Identification of the type of lipid that is elevated is important in the investigation of lipid disorders. Three groups are recognized:

- Hypercholesterolaemia (cholesterol >5.2 mmol l^{-1}) with little elevation of triglyceride;
- Hypertriglyceridaemia (triglyceride >1.8 mmol l^{-1}) with little elevation of cholesterol;
- Combined hyperlipidaemia.

There have been several ways of classifying these disorders and presently the WHO classification (also called the **Fredrickson** system) is widely used. It is based on plasma analysis and there are six categories that have different biochemical profiles, as summarized in *Table 13.3*.

Increased lipid in the serum is seen as a turbid, creamy suspension, and this is characteristic of hyperlipidaemia. Chylomicrons are less dense than the serum and float on the surface of the sample as a creamy layer, rather as cream floats on milk.

Table 13.3 WHO classification of the primary hyperlipidaemias

WHO type	Elevated lipoprotein	Cholesterol	Triglyceride	LDL	HDL	Appearance of serum
Type I	Chylomicrons	N/↑	↑↑	↓	N/↓	Creamy layer
Type IIa	LDL	↑	N	↑	N/↓	Clear
Type IIb	LDL + VLDL	↑	↑	↑	N/↓	Turbid
Type III	IDL	↑	↑	N/↓	N/↓	Turbid
Type IV	VLDL	N/↑	↑	N	N/↓	Turbid + slight creamy layer
Type V	Chylomicrons and VLDL	N/↑	↑↑	N	N/↓	Turbid + thick creamy layer

N, Normal level.

Primary hyperlipidaemias

In the absence of other underlying conditions, the presence of excess levels of lipid in a patient's blood sample is called a primary hyperlipidaemia. There are a number of recognized hyperlipidaemias.

Familial hypercholesterolaemia

This is characterized by elevated cholesterol levels with a normal triglyceride level. The WHO classifies this as a type IIa or IIb hyperlipidaemia. This is a genetic defect of the LDL receptor, with a carrier rate of approximately 1 in 500. Homozygotes usually die from a myocardial infarction before the age of 30. Homozygotes present with the disease in their mid-life with high cholesterol and LDL levels. Symptoms associated with this disease are the deposition of cholesterol in the skin around the eyes (**xanthelasma**) or on tendons (**tendonous xanthomata**). Levels of cholesterol are often >9.0 mmol l^{-1} (see *Box 13.2*).

Box 13.2 Familial hypercholesterolaemia

Joseph Goldstein and Michael Brown shared the Nobel Prize for Physiology and Medicine in 1985 for their work in linking biochemistry, genetics and medicine. They studied patients with familial hypercholesterolaemia, relating high levels of cholesterol with the heart disease these patients developed at an early age. They showed that these patients lacked LDL receptors on their cell surfaces, so that the cholesterol associated with the lipoprotein remained high in the blood, initiating heart disease.

Familial hypertriglyceridaemia

This group of conditions is characterized by an elevated serum triglyceride and VLDL with a normal or slightly raised cholesterol. They are seen as a type IV or V by the WHO classification. In type V, an increase in chylomicrons is also seen. Patients with this condition are at greater risk of an early myocardial infarction and often have triglyceride levels of up to 12.0 mmol l^{-1}.

Familial combined hyperlipidaemia

This condition is the most common of the primary hyperlipidaemias and can present in a number of different ways, falling within different WHO categories. The causes of this condition are not known but it is thought that its inheritance is a dominant trait. Patients with this condition are at a higher risk of developing atherosclerosis.

There are a number of other rare primary hyperlipidaemias and these will not be discussed here.

Secondary hyperlipidaemias

Hyperlipidaemia secondary to other diseases accounts for less than a fifth of all cases. Hypercholesterolaemia is often associated with hypothyroidism and nephrotic syndrome, and hypertriglyceridaemia is associated with alcoholism and diabetes mellitus.

Hypolipidaemia

Hypolipidaemia is a rare condition associated with deficiencies of particular apolipoproteins. **Tangier disease** is a rare autosomal recessive disorder characterized by enhanced catabolism of apo A-1 resulting in low levels of HDL. Hypolipidaemia is also seen in cases of severe malnutrition or malabsorption associated with some types of liver disease.

13.4 ATHEROSCLEROSIS

In modern Western society heart disease is a major cause of death and there is a well-recognized association between heart disease and increased lipid levels (see *Box 13.3*). Atherosclerosis affects the large arteries, often in

---

Box 13.3 Atherosclerosis

At the beginning of the 20th century, it was thought that atherosclerosis was induced by a 'toxic metabolite of animal protein' taken in the diet. In 1912 it was discovered that cholesterol was atherogenic and attention was turned from proteins to lipids in the development of atheroma.

regions of turbulent blood flow found at the sites of arterial junctions. An atherosclerotic plaque is formed by the accumulation of lipid and fibrous deposits in the lining of the artery. These gradually accumulate and occlude the lumen of the artery. Blood flow through the artery gradually diminishes, resulting in the eventual infarction and damage of tissue. Analysis of the atherosclerotic plaque shows that nearly half of the lesion is composed of lipid, mainly cholesterol. It seems that the cholesterol is derived from plasma lipoproteins. The relative levels of LDL and HDL have been shown to be important in assessing the risk of developing atherosclerosis. There is much research showing links between the development of heart disease and the presence of lipid in the blood. The major findings have shown that:

- Increased LDL correlates with **increased** risk of heart disease;
- Increased lipoprotein-(a) correlates with **increased** risk of heart disease;
- Increased HDL correlates with **decreased** risk of heart disease.

Lipoprotein-(a) is a variant of LDL with a higher protein content and is **strongly** associated with the development of atherosclerosis.

Other major factors in developing heart disease are associated with the plasma level of total cholesterol, cigarette smoking and hypertension.

13.5 LABORATORY INVESTIGATIONS OF LIPID

It must be stressed that a **fasting sample** is used, as dietary lipid can invalidate any result. In the investigation of lipids in a blood sample the appearance of the plasma is often useful. *Figure 13.3* shows the appearance of the plasma in the different WHO categories of hyperlipidaemia. If the plasma is clear, the triglyceride is likely to be normal; with high triglyceride levels the plasma is milky in appearance. If the sample is allowed to stand for several hours at 4°C, chylomicrons are seen as a thick creamy layer floating on the top. The presence of chylomicrons with a clear plasma suggests a type I pattern, whereas if the plasma is opaque, then a type V pattern is likely. If the sample has an even, opaque appearance without chylomicrons, it is likely to be a type IV pattern. The most important measurements to be made on the sample are the total cholesterol and total triglyceride levels.

In modern clinical biochemistry laboratories cholesterol and triglyceride levels are measured on large, high-throughput analysers. Enzymatic methods are used which result in a coloured product that is measured spectrophotometrically.

Cholesterol measurements use the enzymes cholesterol esterase and cholesterol oxidase to produce hydrogen peroxide, which can be linked to a number of different reactions that form a coloured product. Hydrogen peroxide can be broken down to oxygen and measured using an oxygen-sensing electrode. The reference range for cholesterol varies depending on the age and gender of the patient and reflects a desired level rather than a range obtained from a healthy population.

Triglyceride measurements utilize the enzyme lipase to form glycerol, and glycerol kinase to produce ADP and glycerol-3-phosphate. Both products

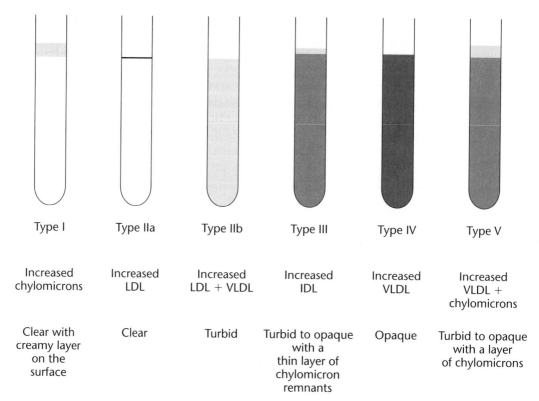

Type I	Type IIa	Type IIb	Type III	Type IV	Type V
Increased chylomicrons	Increased LDL	Increased LDL + VLDL	Increased IDL	Increased VLDL	Increased VLDL + chylomicrons
Clear with creamy layer on the surface	Clear	Turbid	Turbid to opaque with a thin layer of chylomicron remnants	Opaque	Turbid to opaque with a layer of chylomicrons

Figure 13.3
Appearance of the serum in the different categories of the WHO classification of the primary hyperlipidaemias.

can be used in further reactions to produce a coloured or UV-absorbing product. As with cholesterol, the reference range reflects a desired level rather than one obtained from a healthy population.

Lipoprotein analysis can be achieved using electrophoresis and a lipid stain such as Sudan Black or Fast Red. Modern techniques for quantifying individual lipoproteins use antibodies directed against particular apolipo-proteins in an immunoassay.

SUGGESTED FURTHER READING

In addition to relevant chapters in the text books cited in Chapter 1 the following references are recommended.

Hoeg J.M. (1998) Lipoproteins and atherogenesis. *Endocrinology and Metabolism Clinics of North America,* **27**: 569–586.

Kwiterovich Jr, P.O. (2000) The metabolic pathways of high-density lipoprotein, low-density lipoprotein, and triglycerides: a current review. *The American Journal of Cardiology,* **86** (Supplement 1): 5–10.

Moffatt R.J. and Stamford B. (eds) (2005) *Lipid Metabolism and Health*. London: Taylor & Francis Ltd.

Tulenko T.N. and Sumner A.E. (2002) The physiology of lipoproteins. *Journal of Nuclear Cardiology*, **9**: 638–649.

Vance D.E. and Vance J.E. (2002) *Biochemistry of Lipids, Lipoproteins and Membranes*, 4th edition. Oxford: Elsevier.

Yamaguchi Y., Kunitomo M. and Haginaka J. (2002) Assay methods of modified lipoproteins in plasma. *Journal of Chromatography B*, **781**: 313–330.

SELF-ASSESSMENT QUESTIONS

1. In the gut, lipid is digested to what compounds?
2. Which lipoprotein has the highest percentage of triglyceride?
3. What are the major apolipoproteins found in HDL?
4. Where is VLDL synthesized?
5. In which class of hyperlipidaemia does the plasma have a turbid appearance and a thick creamy layer?
6. Which class of hyperlipidaemia is associated with an increased level of IDL?
7. Is Tangier disease associated with hyper- or hypolipidaemia?
8. Which lipoprotein is associated with protection against heart disease?
9. Give three important factors associated with an increased risk of heart disease.

Acid–base balance and blood gases

Learning objectives
After studying this chapter you should confidently be able to:

■ **Describe the mechanisms that control the blood pH.**
Hydrogen ions are generated from sulphur-containing amino acids, phosphorus-containing molecules and from the production of organic acids. The blood pH is regulated by the kidneys (metabolic component) and the lungs (respiratory or non-metabolic component). The normal pH is 7.4, which is equivalent to a hydrogen ion concentration of 40 nmol l^{-1}.

■ **Explain how changes in blood levels of carbon dioxide and bicarbonate affect blood pH.**
There is an equilibrium reaction between hydrogen ions and bicarbonate forming carbonic acid and its dissociation to water and carbon dioxide. This equilibrium reaction can be driven by the enzyme carbonic anhydrase. The respiratory component of acid–base regulation is reflected in the blood pCO_2 and the metabolic component of acid–base regulation is reflected in the blood $[HCO_3^-]$.

■ **Classify the acid–base disorders and describe how compensatory mechanisms restore the pH towards normal.**
An acidosis is the condition where an elevated hydrogen ion concentration is found (a low pH). An alkalosis is the condition where low hydrogen ion concentrations are found (a high pH). An acidosis or alkalosis can be classified as having a metabolic or a respiratory cause. Compensation, whether metabolic or respiratory, attempts to bring the pH back towards normal.

■ **Describe the use of blood gas and other measurements used to investigate acid/base disturbances.**
The measurements of pH, pCO_2 and $[HCO_3^-]$ are performed on arterial blood. The chloride shift is the movement of chloride ions into red blood cells to balance the loss of bicarbonate from the cell and the anion gap is the difference between measured anions and measured cations. Oxygen measurements can aid in the assessment of acid–base disorders.

Everyday living involves burning fuel to supply energy and removing the waste products that can be toxic if left to accumulate. Normal metabolic turnover by the cells will produce an excess of acid which is, in fact, hydrogen ions produced in the cell. If the hydrogen ions are not removed, their accumulation and the consequent rise in acidity within the cell will eventually lead to cell death. In this chapter we shall see how acid is formed and transported in the blood to sites of excretion.

Acidity of a fluid is measured by **pH**, which is inversely related to the log of **hydrogen ion** concentration (see *Box 14.1*). Low pH (high hydrogen ion concentration) values are given by acidic solutions, whereas alkaline solutions have high pH values (low hydrogen ion concentration). In health the pH of the body is very tightly regulated and enzymes work at optimum pH values. If the pH of a cell, or of the body, changes significantly an acid–base disturbance occurs, leading to pathological symptoms and eventually, if left untreated, to death.

Box 14.1 Invention of the pH scale

Sören Sörensen (1868–1939) invented the pH scale for measuring acidity in 1909 at the Carlsberg Laboratory in Copenhagen.

A number of metabolic pathways contribute to the production of hydrogen ions within the cell. The most important are:

■ Oxidation of sulphur-containing amino acids giving sulphuric acid, H_2SO_4;
■ The hydrolysis of phosphorus-containing proteins and lipids giving phosphoric acid, H_3PO_4;
■ The production of ketoacids and lactic acid from carbohydrate metabolism.

Approximately 40–80 mmol of the above acids are produced every day, mainly from the breakdown of dietary protein.

To maintain careful control of the pH the body has a sophisticated buffering mechanism. The three most important buffer systems are:

■ The bicarbonate system;
■ Proteins, mainly haemoglobin;
■ The phosphate system.

These buffer systems are important because they mop up excess hydrogen ions produced by the cell. Of these, the bicarbonate buffering system is the most important, making up approximately three-quarters of the body's buffering capacity. Hydrogen ions combine with bicarbonate ions to form carbonic acid, which itself dissociates to water and carbon dioxide. Some cells contain an enzyme, **carbonic anhydrase**, which catalyses this reaction. These reactions are shown below:

$$H^+A^- + Na^+HCO_3^- \leftrightarrow Na^+A^- + H_2CO_3 \leftrightarrow H_2O + CO_2$$

The reaction is driven to the right, which means that hydrogen ions, produced in cells and buffered by the bicarbonate system, generate carbon dioxide and reduce available bicarbonate. Uncontrolled generation of hydrogen ions would lead to high blood levels of dissolved carbon dioxide and low levels of bicarbonate ions. Fortunately there are mechanisms which remove hydrogen ions and maintain blood pH within very tight limits.

14.1   CONTROL OF pH

Two organs control the pH of the body: the **lungs** and the **kidneys**. In health, the hydrogen ions from non-volatile and organic acids are removed by the kidneys into the urine, and carbon dioxide, from the breakdown of carbonic acid, is excreted by the lungs. The blood transports acidic waste products from the site of production in the tissues to the sites of excretion, namely the kidneys and lungs. These two excretory pathways form two components of acid–base metabolism. The lungs represent and control the **respiratory component** of acid–base balance and the kidneys represent and control the **metabolic component**. It is the interaction and balance of these two systems that controls the pH of the body, and diseases affecting either of these two organs can affect the acid–base balance, giving rise to an abnormal pH.

Respiratory control

The lungs are responsible for **gas exchange**, giving oxygen to the red blood cells and removing carbon dioxide (effectively removing acid) (see *Fig. 14.1*). In the tissues carbon dioxide is produced and diffuses into erythrocytes where it combines with water to form bicarbonate ions and hydrogen ions. This process is under the influence of carbonic anhydrase. Deoxygenated haemoglobin is reduced by hydrogen ions, acting as a buffer. As bicarbonate ions diffuse out of the cell, chloride ions diffuse in to restore electrical neutrality; this is known as the **chloride shift**. In the lungs the reverse reaction occurs and reduced haemoglobin absorbs fresh oxygen, releasing hydrogen ions, which combine with bicarbonate under the influence of carbonic anhydrase to produce water and carbon dioxide. Carbon dioxide diffuses rapidly into the alveolus and is exhaled. The erythrocytes return to the tissues in the arterial blood that is oxygenated.

Metabolic control

The kidneys are the site where hydrogen ions are excreted and also where bicarbonate is generated. Blood is filtered in the glomerulus to produce the glomerular filtrate, which contains small proteins and dissolved cations and anions, including acid anions such as sulphate and phosphate. *Figure 14.2* illustrates three mechanisms by which hydrogen ions are excreted into the urine. In the kidney's tubular cells, the enzyme carbonic anhydrase catalyses the reaction between carbon and water to form bicarbonate and hydrogen ions. Bicarbonate ions diffuse from the cell into the blood and hydrogen ions are transported into the kidney tubule; this process has the effect of generating bicarbonate ions. In the kidney tubule there are two main buffer

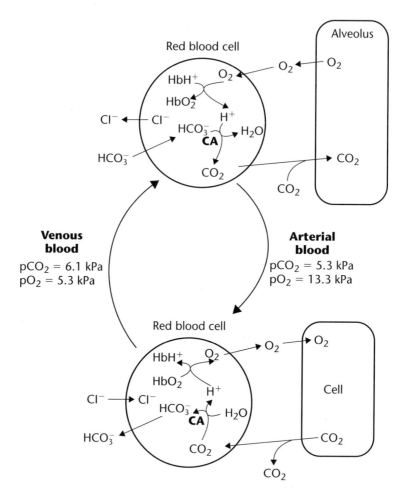

Figure 14.1
The excretion of carbon dioxide generated within respiring cells and transported in the blood to be lost through the lungs. CA = carbonic anhydrase; Hb, haemoglobin.

systems, which remove the excreted hydrogen ions. Pathway A shown in *Fig. 14.2* leads to the generation of ammonium ions from ammonia, mainly derived from glutamine. Pathway B shows the buffering capacity of phosphate via the generation of sodium dihydrogen phosphate. These two pathways occur in the distal tubular cells and the buffering capacity depends somewhat on the amount of phosphate and ammonia excreted. The third pathway shown in *Fig. 14.2*, pathway C, involves the reabsorption of bicarbonate ions filtered from the blood. In this case hydrogen ions are exchanged for sodium ions in the glomerular filtrate, a process achieved via a sodium pump.

The kidney tubule is lined with cells containing carbonic anhydrase in the brush border of the tubule lumen. Carbon dioxide and water are generated from the enzymatic reaction between excreted hydrogen ions and bicar-

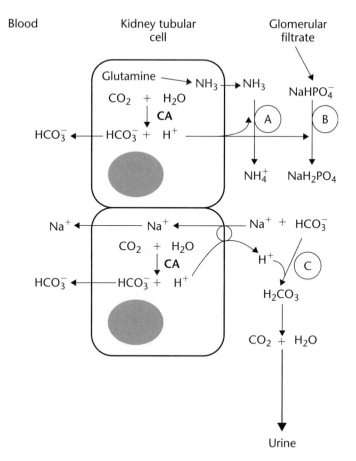

Figure 14.2
The excretion of hydrogen ions by the kidney. See text for a detailed description of
the pathways A, B, and C. CA = carbonic anhydrase.

bonate in the glomerular filtrate. The carbon dioxide diffuses into the
tubular cells and reacts with water, under the influence of intracellular
carbonic anhydrase, to reform bicarbonate, which diffuses from the cells
into the blood. These reactions, catalysed by carbonic anhydrase in two
different sites, effectively bring about the reabsorption of bicarbonate ions
from the glomerular filtrate.

14.2 NORMAL pH

The normal pH of the body is 7.4. This can be calculated from the
Henderson–Hasselbalch equation using constants for bicarbonate buffers:

$$pH = 6.1 + \log_{10} [HCO_3^-] / [H_2CO_3]$$

where 6.1 is the pH of the bicarbonate buffer system and the square
brackets indicate molar concentration.

From the above equation we can see that:

$$pH \propto [HCO_3^-] / [H_2CO_3] \qquad (1)$$

We have seen earlier that bicarbonate forms carbon dioxide, which dissolves in the body's water. The amount of carbon dioxide in the blood is related to its partial pressure (pCO_2), which can be measured using a carbon dioxide electrode (see later in the chapter). The relationship below is found:

$$[H_2CO_3] = pCO_2 \times 0.2295 \qquad (2)$$

where pCO_2 is measured in kPa (kilopascals). (Some older textbooks still use mmHg as the unit of partial pressure and, in this case, 0.0306 is used as the multiplier in the above equation.)

Combining (1) and (2) we obtain:

$$pH \propto [HCO_3^-] / [pCO_2]$$

This shows that the pH is related to the bicarbonate concentration and pCO_2. pH is inversely related to the hydrogen ion concentration and so the above relationship could be written as:

$$[H^+] \propto pCO_2 / [HCO_3^-] \qquad (3)$$

In health the pH of the blood is **7.4**, which is equivalent to a hydrogen ion concentration of **40 nmol l^{-1}**. To maintain this value the ratio of bicarbonate concentration to pCO_2 is kept constant (see *Box 14.2*). This means that in order to restore normal pH from a low pH (high $[H^+]$) either the pCO_2 will need to be lowered or the $[HCO_3^-]$ needs to be raised. Conversely, when the pH is high (low $[H^+]$) the pCO_2 has to be raised or $[HCO_3^-]$ lowered to restore the pH to normal. The reference range for pCO_2 is 4.5–6.0 kPa, whilst that for $[HCO_3^-]$ is 20–30 mmol l^{-1}. Referring to equation (3) above, we can say that **pCO_2 is the respiratory component** and **$[HCO_3^-]$ is the metabolic component**.

Box 14.2 Hydrogen ion concentration

The hydrogen ion concentration of a fluid of pH 7.4 is

$$7.4 = \log_{10} 1/[H^+] = -\log_{10} [H^+]$$
$$[H^+] = 10^{-7.4} = 3.98 \times 10^{-8} \text{ moles}$$
$$= 40 \text{ nM } (40 \text{ nmol l}^{-1})$$

14.3   DISORDERS OF ACID–BASE BALANCE

As we have seen above, the pH of the blood is tightly controlled by the lungs and kidneys, maintaining a pH of 7.4. In health, if the pH changes due to normal physiological activity such as strenuous exercise, it is rapidly restored to normal. Problems arise when the normal mechanisms are unable to cope with changes of pH. There are two primary causes of this:

- A prolonged production of hydrogen ions or prolonged loss of hydrogen ions too great for the normal mechanisms to accommodate;
- Disease of the lungs or kidneys which prevents the normal compensation mechanisms from functioning effectively.

Disorders of acid–base balance are broadly grouped as an **acidosis** or an **alkalosis** depending on whether there is a general accumulation of hydrogen ions, an acidosis (low pH), or if there is a loss of hydrogen ions, an alkalosis (high pH). These are both further subdivided into two more groups depending on the cause of the disorder. If the pH imbalance is due to metabolic or renal disease, it is classified as 'metabolic' and where the problem is due to lung function, it is classified as respiratory.

Knowing the $[HCO_3^-]$ and pCO_2 enables classification of the acid–base disorder. **Remember**:

$$[H^+] \propto pCO_2 / [HCO_3^-]$$

and that PCO_2 reflects respiratory activity and $[HCO_3^-]$ reflects metabolic activity.

The four main acid–base disorders are:

1. **Metabolic acidosis**, an accumulation of hydrogen ions resulting in a decreased bicarbonate concentration.

$$[H^+] \propto pCO_2 / [HCO_3^-]$$
$$\uparrow \qquad \qquad \downarrow$$

2. **Respiratory acidosis**, an excess of hydrogen ions due to insufficient gas exchange resulting in increased pCO_2:

$$[H^+] \propto pCO_2 / [HCO_3^-]$$
$$\uparrow \qquad \uparrow$$

3. **Metabolic alkalosis**, a decrease in hydrogen ion concentration resulting in an elevated bicarbonate concentration:

$$[H^+] \propto pCO_2 / [HCO_3^-]$$
$$\downarrow \qquad \qquad \uparrow$$

4. **Respiratory alkalosis**, a decrease in hydrogen ion concentration due to excessive gas exchange resulting in lowered pCO_2:

$$[H^+] \propto pCO_2 / [HCO_3^-]$$
$$\downarrow \qquad \downarrow$$

Compensation

It is important to realize that in conditions which disturb the acid–base balance by an overproduction of acid or an excessive loss of acid, there is a compensation mechanism that tries to restore the pH. This is because both lungs and kidneys are involved in maintaining blood pH. Where lung function is causing the acid–base disturbance, the kidney increases its excretion of hydrogen ions in an attempt to restore blood pH. This is known as **renal compensation**. Where the acid–base disorder is due to a metabolic problem or renal insufficiency, the lungs can offer some compensation by adjusting the rate of gas exchange, i.e. the rate of carbon dioxide loss. This is known as **respiratory compensation**. If the compensation mechanism restores the pH to within the reference range, this is a **fully compensated** disorder. In this case the pH is normal but pCO_2 and $[HCO_3^-]$ are grossly abnormal. **Partial compensation** is when the pH has not been fully restored to normal.

14.4 PATHOPHYSIOLOGY

Disorders of acid–base balance can be divided into acidosis and alkalosis, each having a metabolic and a respiratory origin.

Metabolic acidosis – low $[HCO_3^-]$

This is due to:

■ Increased production of acid;
■ Decreased excretion of acid;
■ Excessive loss of bicarbonate ions.

Increased acid production is seen in metabolic disease where there is an excess production of organic acids, for example ketoacids seen in diabetes mellitus, or lactic acid seen in cases of lactic acidosis. Kidney disease and cases of mineralocorticoid deficiency result in a reduction in excretion of acid from the kidneys and accumulation of acid in the blood. Excess acid is buffered by bicarbonate, resulting in reduced bicarbonate concentration and a lower pH. In cases of acute diarrhoea or drainage from a pancreatic fistula, there is a loss of bicarbonate, resulting in an altered ratio with pCO_2 and consequently a lowered pH.

The high levels of hydrogen ions (low pH):

■ Impair cardiac muscle contraction with the possibility of cardiac failure;
■ Exchange with potassium in cells leading to **hyperkalaemia**;
■ Enhance mobilization of calcium from bones, thereby decreasing binding of calcium to proteins and calcium reabsorption by the kidney. In prolonged acidosis there can be a generalized loss of calcium from the body and there may be formation of kidney stones.

Compensation of metabolic acidosis is achieved through the respiratory pathway. Respiratory compensation removes more carbon dioxide through the lungs, achieved by **hyperventilation**. This lowers the pCO_2 and restores the pCO_2 : $[HCO_3^-]$ ratio and hence the pH. Respiratory compensation rarely returns pH to normal.

Respiratory acidosis – high pCO$_2$

This is due to:

- Decreased respiration rate;
- Decreased gas exchange due to lung disease.

A decreased respiration rate can result from depression of the central nervous system following infections, tumours, trauma or from drug overdoses. Neuromuscular disease such as polio or multiple sclerosis and instances of physical restriction or injury to the chest can affect respiratory efficiency. Decreased gas exchange is seen in respiratory infections such as pneumonia and bronchitis or where there is oedema or a foreign body obstruction.

High levels of carbon dioxide in the blood (**hypercapnia**) would normally stimulate the central nervous system to induce hyperventilation to lower the pCO$_2$. When this cannot occur, the high pCO$_2$ causes cerebral vasodilation, leading to headache, drowsiness, stupor and coma.

Compensation of respiratory acidosis occurs through the kidney excreting more acid and generating more bicarbonate, thereby restoring the pCO$_2$: [HCO$_3^-$] ratio.

Metabolic alkalosis – high [HCO$_3^-$]

This is due to:

- Loss of hydrogen ions and subsequent overproduction of bicarbonate;
- Ingestion or infusion of bicarbonate.

Excessive hydrogen ion loss can be from the gastrointestinal tract or the kidney. Excessive and prolonged vomiting or diarrhoea can lead to loss of hydrogen ions. Vomiting of stomach contents and fluids leads to loss of hydrochloric acid, and the body generates an excess of bicarbonate as a result of replacing the lost hydrogen ions. Renal losses of hydrogen ions are seen in those patients with a mineralocorticoid excess and those taking thiazide diuretics. Rarely, a metabolic alkalosis can be induced from the ingestion of bicarbonate, but an adult would need to take over 1 mole of bicarbonate to influence blood pH. An overenthusiastic self-administration of antacid therapy can lead to a metabolic alkalosis, especially if taken with milk; this unusual condition is known as **milk-alkali syndrome**.

High blood pH causes:

- Ionization of calcium ions, lowering the ionized fraction causing increased neuromuscular activity;
- Hypokalaemia as a result of the exchange of cellular hydrogen ions for blood potassium ions;
- Suppression of the respiratory centres, thereby allowing compensation by **hypoventilation** and reducing CO$_2$ loss and thus acid loss. This mechanism is countered by the resulting hypoxia stimulating the respiratory centre and respiratory rate. This has the effect of raising the pCO$_2$ and restoring the pCO$_2$: [HCO$_3^-$] ratio.

Respiratory alkalosis – low pCO_2

This is due to stimulation of the respiratory rate.

Overbreathing (hyperventilation) results in excessive loss of carbon dioxide and therefore loss of hydrogen ions. This can result from stimulation of the respiratory centres by drugs such as salicylate, hypoxaemia or by anxiety or hysteria. Other conditions such as infection, trauma or tumours may also affect the respiratory centre.

Hypocapnia (low blood carbon dioxide level) leads to cerebral vasoconstriction and the feeling of light-headedness.

Compensation of respiratory alkalosis is achieved by lowering bicarbonate levels by the retention of hydrogen ions by the kidney, thus restoring the $pCO_2 : [HCO_3^-]$ ratio.

Mixed acid–base disturbances

The acid–base disorders described above are termed **simple disorders**, indicating a single cause and compensatory mechanism. In approximately 40% of cases, the acid–base disorder is a **mixed disorder** arising from a combination of simple disorders. An example of a combination of metabolic and respiratory acidosis resulting in a severe acidaemia would be: a very low pH, an increased pCO_2 and a low $[HCO_3^-]$.

14.5 ANION GAP

To aid in the investigation of an acid–base disorder, a useful measurement is the **anion gap**. This is the difference (in mmol) between the **measured anions** (sodium and potassium) and **measured cations** (chloride and bicarbonate). The normal anion gap is:

$$(140 + 4) - (100 + 27) = 17$$
$$\quad \text{Na} \quad \text{K} \qquad \text{Cl}^- \quad HCO_3^- \quad \text{(measured in mmol l}^{-1})$$

The figure of 17 is due to unmeasured anions; theoretically there is a net zero difference when all the anions and cations are taken into account. The term 'anion gap' should technically be called the unmeasured anions. The anion gap is useful in determining the cause of an acidosis. If there is an excess of lactic or keto acids, the additional anions (lactate or keto anions), which are not measured, replace the bicarbonate consumed by the excess hydrogen ions, giving an increased anion gap. In cases of acidosis caused by loss of bicarbonate, for example with diarrhoea, chloride ions replace the bicarbonate and the anion gap remains normal.

14.6 BLOOD GASES

Carbon dioxide is transported in the erythrocytes and gas exchange occurs in the lungs. Oxygen is the life-giving gas that is also exchanged in the lungs and transported in the erythrocytes. The amount of oxygen in the blood is related to the measured partial pressure of oxygen (pO_2). Haemoglobin is the protein found within the erythrocyte that is responsible for carrying oxygen. When fully saturated, 1 g of haemoglobin can carry 1.34 ml of oxygen. At pO_2 levels greater than 10.5 kPa the haemoglobin is virtually saturated with oxygen (see *Box 14.3*).

Box 14.3 Haemoglobin

The structure of haemoglobin was deduced by Max Perutz in 1953 using X-ray crystallography. His colleague John Kendrew worked out the structure of myoglobin, a related protein. For their work in this field they shared the Nobel Prize for Chemistry in 1962.

When acid–base studies are carried out in the clinical laboratory it is usual to measure the blood gases and the haemoglobin level at the same time. Carbon dioxide levels are used in acid–base assessment, and oxygen levels can help in the evaluation of the pathology surrounding the acid–base disturbance. Blood gases are measured on arterial blood, and in health the normal pO_2 level is 11–15 kPa (see *Box 14.4*). Assuming normal haemoglobin levels, the pO_2 can give useful information about respiratory function. Low levels of pO_2 (<8 kPa) are seen in those patients where there is respiratory insufficiency. A low pO_2 with a low pCO_2 is seen in those patients who are hypoventilating, as insufficient oxygen is being passed into the blood and carbon dioxide is not being removed. This picture is often found in those patients with mechanical defects to the lung which prevent adequate respiratory function. As carbon dioxide diffuses and dissolves in fluid much more rapidly than oxygen, the situation where there is a low pO_2 and a normal or low pCO_2 indicates a sufficient blood supply to the lungs, as carbon dioxide is not accumulating, but inadequate perfusion of oxygen as a result of lung pathology. This leads to the accumulation of fluid, preventing adequate oxygen diffusion.

Box 14.4 Units of pressure

In many books the unit of pressure is given as mmHg, where 1 mmHg is 0.1333 kPa. Thus, a pO_2 of 90 mmHg is equivalent to 12 kPa.

14.7 BLOOD GAS MEASUREMENTS

In modern clinical biochemistry laboratories blood gas measurements and pH measurements are performed on a single arterial blood sample by a dedicated instrument. These instruments are often sited on high-dependency units such as intensive care and cardiac units. The measurement of blood gases is often required as an urgent investigation. The instrument has three electrodes that are used in the measurement procedure, measuring pH, pCO_2 and pO_2, and from these measurements the bicarbonate is calculated using formulae based on the Henderson–Hasselbalch equation seen earlier in this chapter.

The pH electrode is basically a glass electrode that is selective for hydrogen ions, generating a voltage across the glass membrane. The measured voltage is related to the pH by the **Nernst** equation.

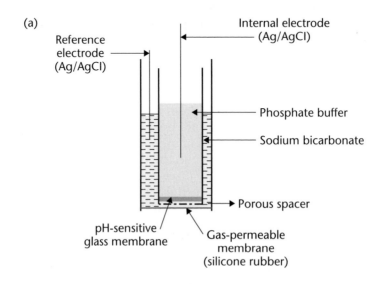

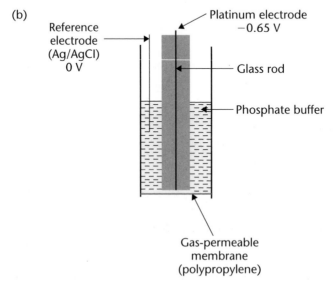

Figure 14.3
Illustrations showing (a) a CO_2 electrode and (b) an oxygen electrode. See text for the principle of operation of these two types of electrode.

The carbon dioxide electrode has a gas-permeable membrane made from silicon rubber that allows the gas to diffuse into a thin film of sodium bicarbonate solution. Carbon dioxide dissolves in the solution, changing the pH, which is monitored by a pH electrode. These measurements are **voltammetric**, relying on the measurement of voltage changes by the electrode. *Figure 14.3a* illustrates a carbon dioxide electrode; the pH electrode with its hydrogen ion selective membrane is shown immersed in sodium bicarbonate. The voltage generated across the membrane is measured against the silver/silver chloride reference electrode.

The oxygen electrode, in contrast to the other two electrodes, is an **amperometric** device that measures the amount of current flowing between two electrodes. In the oxygen electrode a gas-permeable membrane made from polypropylene allows oxygen to pass into a solution of phosphate buffer. The cathode is a platinum wire with a potential of –0.65 V. Oxygen from the sample is reduced at the electrode surface, allowing current flow, which is measured. Higher oxygen levels in the sample result in a greater current flow at the electrode. *Figure 14.3b* shows a diagram of an oxygen electrode. Oxygen electrodes are not only found in blood gas analysers but are also used in conjunction with enzyme reactions where oxygen is used or generated by the reaction. A common application for oxygen electrodes is in electrochemical methods for measuring glucose.

SUGGESTED FURTHER READING

In addition to relevant chapters in the textbooks cited in Chapter 1, the following review articles are recommended.

Dubose T. and Hamm L. (2002) *Acid-Base and Electrolyte Disorders: A Companion to Brenner and Rector's The Kidney.* Philadelphia: W.B. Saunders.

Durward A. and Murdoch I. (2003) Understanding acid–base balance. *Current Paediatrics*, **13**: 513–519.

Feld L.G. (2001) *Handbook of Fluid, Electrolyte and Acid-base Disorders.* London: Butterworth-Heinemann Ltd.

Kulpmann W.-R., Stummvoll H.-K. and Lehmann P. (2006) *Electrolytes, Acid-base Balance and Blood Gases.* Heidelberg: Springer-Verlag.

SELF-ASSESSMENT QUESTIONS

1. How is pH related to the hydrogen ion concentration?
2. What is the most important buffer system involved in acid–base balance?
3. Which organ is associated with the metabolic control of acid–base balance?
4. Blood pH is proportional to which two blood parameters?
5. What is the underlying biochemical change seen in metabolic acidosis?

6. What is the underlying biochemical change seen in respiratory alkalosis?
7. How is the compensation of a metabolic alkalosis brought about?
8. How is the compensation of a respiratory acidosis brought about?
9. A patient was found to have a slightly low to normal pH, a high pCO_2 and high $[HCO_3^-]$. What type of acid–base disturbance was present?
10. What is the fundamental difference between the principle of the carbon dioxide electrode and the oxygen electrode?

Immunoglobulins

> ## Learning objectives
> *After studying this chapter you should confidently be able to:*
>
> ■ **Describe the classification and structure of antibodies.**
> Antibodies are immunoglobulins (also called gammaglobulins) and are
> secreted by plasma cells. There are five antibody isotypes: IgG, IgA, IgM,
> IgD and IgE. An antibody derived from a single clone of cells is called a
> monoclonal antibody. Pooled antibody from many clones is called
> polyclonal antibody. Antibodies bind specifically to a particular antigen.
>
> ■ **Briefly outline the biochemical changes seen in monoclonal
> gammopathies.**
> Hypergammaglobulinaemia is an abnormal excess of antibody in the
> blood. Hypogammaglobulinaemia is an abnormal deficit of antibody in
> the blood. Monoclonal gammopathies involve the production of a
> monoclonal antibody. Monoclonal antibody separates as a single band by
> agarose electrophoresis, called a paraprotein.
>
> ■ **Explain the principles behind immunoprecipitation and
> immunoblotting techniques.**
> Individual antibody concentrations can be measured by
> immunoprecipitation techniques. Paraprotein typing can be performed
> using immunofixation. Both these techniques involve the formation of an
> insoluble immunoprecipitate, which is formed by the action of a specific
> antibody directed against the component being measured (IgG, IgM,
> etc.).

In this section we shall look at conditions that affect the body's ability to
defend itself against pathogenic organisms. To maintain health, the body
requires a system to combat these organisms and this is the **immune system**.
The immune system can be divided into two parts: one which recognizes
specific pathogens or foreign proteins, and the other which demonstrates a
non-specific response to infection. The former is the **acquired immune
system** and is considered in this chapter; the latter is the **innate immune
system** and is discussed in the next chapter.

The acquired immune system consists of a complex interaction of specialized cells (macrophages, B lymphocytes and T lymphocytes) producing a

vast array of soluble products. These soluble products fall into two categories: (1) messengers called cytokines, responsible for activation, differentiation and proliferation of cells; and (2) those products (called antibodies) which interact and bind specifically to foreign material, thereby aiding its neutralization and elimination. An important role of the clinical biochemistry department is the analysis, both qualitative and quantitative, of serum and urine samples for antibodies. Abnormalities, both in the amount and in the distribution of antibody types, can indicate a disease process that may result in the patient not being able to mount an adequate defence against infectious agents.

15.1 ANTIBODIES

Serum proteins separated by electrophoresis can be classified according to their migration. The major protein bands are albumin, which moves the furthest, followed by the α, β and γ bands (see *Fig. 12.1*). Antibodies migrate in the **gamma** region of the electrophoresis strip and are thus sometimes called **gammaglobulins**. Antibodies are more accurately named immunoglobulins and are synthesized by the immune system in response to material foreign to the body such as bacteria, viruses or toxins. The body recognizes the substance as foreign and, through a complicated interaction of cells, B lymphocytes are stimulated to differentiate into **plasma cells**, which then synthesize and secrete antibody. These interactions take place in the spleen and lymph nodes and the antibody released is eventually distributed throughout the body by the lymphatic and circulatory systems (see *Box 15.1*).

Box 15.1 Antibodies and antigens

The presence of 'agents' in the blood which could neutralize toxins had been postulated from the 1890s, with work by Paul Ehrlich, Emil von Behring, Karl Landsteiner, Robert Koch and Jules Bordet being the most important. It was during this time that the terms antibody and antigen were introduced. Other terms were used for antibodies that described particular aspects of their properties – for example, agglutinins, precipitins and opsonins.

It was not until the 1930s that Michael Heidelberger and Forrest Kendall produced a purified antibody preparation from horse serum. Studies on antibody preparations by Theodor Svedberg, Arne Tiselius and Elvin Kabat determined the molecular weight and showed that antibodies belonged to the globulin fraction with slow electrophoretic mobility.

Despite all that was known about antibodies, it was not until the late 1960s that the structure of the antibody molecule was deduced when it was realized that the protein produced in multiple myeloma was a structurally homogenous protein. Gerald Edelman and Rodney Porter studied the structure of immunoglobulins, showing the protein to be made of heavy and light chains held together by disulphide bridges and determining that there were two antigen-binding sites, allowing agglutination to take place. Edelman sequenced the molecule and with other known information Porter deduced the Y-shaped structure of IgG. Edelman and Porter were awarded a Nobel Prize in 1972 for their work on antibody structure.

The basic antibody structure is shown in *Fig. 15.1* and consists of two identical pairs of protein chains. The two longer chains are called heavy chains and have a molecular weight of 50 kilodaltons (kDa); the shorter chains are called light chains with a molecular weight of about 25 kDa. There are five types of heavy chain, each given the name of a Greek letter, and these form the different antibody **isotypes**. The type of heavy chain making the antibody gives rise to the antibody class (isotype); for example, antibody with γ chains is called immunoglobulin G (IgG). There are two types of light chain found, called kappa (κ) light chains and lambda (λ) light chains. The light chains of any one antibody molecule will be either kappa light chains *or* lambda light chains, but *never* both, and thus an individual antibody is classified by its heavy and light chain. *Table 15.1* lists the isotypes of antibodies, their defining heavy chain, the number of units in the structure and their most important attribute.

The substance to which an antibody binds is called an **antigen**. A given antibody will bind only to a specific antigen. It is this specificity that makes antibodies unique in their action, and this can be exploited in immuno-diagnostics and immunotherapeutics. Antibodies have at least two antigen-binding sites, and as a consequence they are able to crosslink large antigens to form a large, insoluble complex called an **immune complex** or **immuno-precipitate**. By binding to antigen and forming an immune complex, the foreign material (the antigen) is rendered harmless and removed from the body. Besides neutralizing and removing foreign material, antibodies are

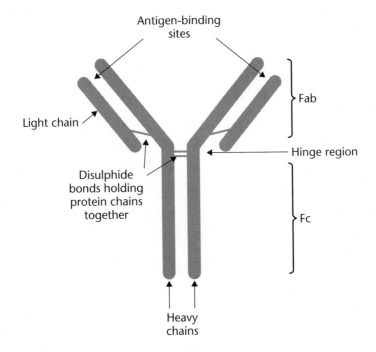

Figure 15.1
The basic structure of an antibody.

Table 15.1 The antibodies

Immunoglobulin name	Heavy chain	Structure	Important attribute
Immunoglobulin G (IgG)	γ	Monomer	Most common antibody in body fluids
Immunoglobulin M (IgM)	μ	Pentamer	First antibody to be synthesized
Immunoglobulin A (IgA)	α	Dimer	Found in secretions
Immunoglobulin D (IgD)	δ	Monomer	Found on young B lymphocytes
Immunoglobulin E (IgE)	ε	Monomer	Involved in allergy

also important in the activation of complement (see next chapter) and aiding phagocytosis. *Table 15.2* gives a summary of the biological functions attributed to the three most abundant classes of antibody found in serum.

Antibodies are synthesized to react with specific antigens: one B cell will give rise to one antibody with a particular specificity, i.e. it will only bind to a single antigen. If a particular B cell is stimulated to synthesize antibody, then that cell will divide and proliferate, producing a clone of cells, all identical and all producing antibody of the same specificity. An antibody produced from a single clone of B cells is called a **monoclonal antibody**. If many different B cells are stimulated to synthesize antibody, many clones of B cells are formed. Antibody produced by many clones of B cells is called **polyclonal antibody** and is made of many hundreds or thousands of clones. The normal immune response to an infection or to a foreign material is to activate many B cell clones to produce polyclonal antibodies. A few individuals produce an oligoclonal (a few clones being activated) or a monoclonal response. Usually the presence of a monoclonal antibody in the blood, particularly at high concentrations, is the result of a pathological process (see *Box 15.2*).

Table 15.2 Functions associated with the three major antibody classes

	IgG	IgM	IgA
Blood concentration (g l^{-1})	5.0–13.5	0.5–2.5	0.5–3.5
Molecular weight (kDa)	150	900	400
Agglutinates bacteria	+	+	+
Neutralizes viruses	+	–	–
Neutralizes toxins	+	–	–
Activates complement	+	++	–
Aids phagocytosis	+	+	–
Crosses the placenta	+	–	–
Secreted antibody	–	–	+

> **Box 15.2 Immunoglobulin reference ranges**
>
> Reference ranges for the immunoglobulins in plasma in adults:
>
> IgG   5–13.5 g l^{-1}
> IgA   0.5–3.5 g l^{-1}
> IgM   0.5–2.5 g l^{-1}
> IgD   <0.1 g l^{-1}
> IgE   <0.005 g l^{-1}

15.2 DISORDERS ASSOCIATED WITH ANTIBODIES

There are two types of disorder associated with antibodies that require investigation by the clinical biochemistry laboratory. There are those conditions where an excessive amount of antibody is being produced inappropriately, and other conditions where insufficient antibody is produced. An excess amount of antibody in the blood is called **hypergammaglobulinaemia**, whereas insufficient antibody is called **hypogammaglobulinaemia** (here 'gamma' refers to the region of migration of antibodies during electrophoresis).

Hypergammaglobulinaemia

Increased levels of antibody in the blood can be a result of an increased polyclonal or monoclonal antibody production. Increased levels of total immunoglobulin (a polyclonal increase) are seen in many conditions, usually as a response to a chronic infection or an autoimmune disease (where the body mistakes a tissue as being foreign and starts to synthesize antibody against that tissue, which is then destroyed by the immune system).

If a clone of B cells becomes large then the antibody it produces becomes a significant proportion of the total and can be seen as a discrete band in the gamma region of an electrophoresis strip. This monoclonal immunoglobulin is often called a **paraprotein**. In this case there is an overproduction of a single antibody isotype and conditions that lead to this situation are known as **monoclonal gammopathies**. These conditions involve the uncontrolled proliferation of a single clone of B cells or plasma cells and, as such, they can be thought of as a neoplastic disease of these cells. There are three main monoclonal gammopathies:

■ Multiple myeloma;
■ Macroglobulinaemia;
■ Heavy-chain disease.

Multiple myeloma

Multiple myeloma is a malignant condition where a single clone of B cells produces an excess of monoclonal antibody (paraprotein). The malignancy spreads to the bones, giving characteristic bone lesions seen on X-ray. Often the first symptoms are of bone pain or low back pain. In 50% of the cases, the cells produce an excess of light chains that are small enough to be filtered in the kidney and appear in the urine as **Bence–Jones** protein. The antibody produced can be of any class although some types of monoclonal antibody are more common than others. Approximately 20% of patients produce only light chains. *Table 15.3* gives the frequency of the different classes of antibody found in multiple myeloma.

As more 'abnormal' monoclonal antibody is produced, normal bone marrow function is impaired and fewer red cells, white cells, and platelets are formed. Normal antibody production is also suppressed, resulting in the patient becoming anaemic and more susceptible to infections. Very high levels of paraprotein in the blood cause an increase in the viscosity of the blood, i.e. the blood becomes thicker and the heart is therefore put under stress.

Table 15.3 Approximate frequency of antibody classes found in patients with multiple myeloma

Antibody class	Frequency (percentage)
IgG	53
IgA	25
IgD	2
IgM	0.5
IgE	<0.1
Light chains only	20

Macroglobulinaemia

This is also known as **Waldenström's macroglobulinaemia** and is associated with the production of excessive amounts of IgM. This high molecular weight protein causes the blood to have increased viscosity, leading to slower blood flow. Other symptoms include neurological changes, bleeding and decreased synthesis of the other immunoglobulins, ultimately leading to hypogammaglobulinaemia.

Heavy-chain disease

Also known as **Franklin's disease**, this rare condition is characterized by a paraprotein that has a molecular weight of approximately 55 kDa, the same weight as immunoglobulin heavy chains.

Hypogammaglobulinaemia

Low levels of immunoglobulin arise as a result of impaired synthesis. If the levels fall too far, the immune system is impaired and the patient becomes susceptible to infections. Physiological hypogammaglobulinaemia is seen in newborn infants before their immune system starts to produce IgG and IgA. Otherwise it is the result of a pathological process, which may be due to genetic disease or acquired conditions. In genetic conditions there is an inability to synthesize antibody. This may be a single class of antibody or it may be a complete absence of antibody; an example of this is Burton's X-linked agammaglobulinopathy. Acquired conditions result if a deficiency in the materials required to synthesize antibody occurs, such as happens in malnutrition, or if there is a loss of cells controlling the synthesis of antibody. In cases of human immunodeficiency virus (HIV) infections, the cells which control the immune response are destroyed, resulting in falling levels of antibody production.

Hypogammaglobulinaemia is seen in patients undergoing immunosuppressive therapy and in patients with malignancy. Paradoxically, patients with an overproduction of a monoclonal antibody can show suppression of normal antibody production, leading to hypogammaglobulinaemia.

15.3 LABORATORY INVESTIGATION OF ANTIBODIES

The laboratory investigation of antibodies involves two types of investigation. First, an assessment of total antibody can be made, and secondly, an assessment of the individual antibody isotypes can be made. The assessment can involve both qualitative and quantitative studies.

Total antibody

The total antibody concentration in a blood sample can give a quick guide to the immune status of a patient. This measurement can be a very rough indication obtained by subtracting the albumin concentration from the total protein, giving the globulin concentration. This is really only a screening method – where a high globulin concentration is found, further investigations are performed to identify why the globulin fraction is elevated. Electrophoresis followed by **scanning densitometry** can be used to give a more accurate estimation of total antibody concentration and, in addition, the presence of a monoclonal band in the gamma region can be identified. *Figure 15.2* shows a paraprotein band on an electrophoresis strip. Electrophoresis does not identify which type of antibody is giving rise to this monoclonal band, and so further investigations into the individual antibody concentrations and types must be undertaken.

Antibody isotypes

In the laboratory investigation into the antibody isotypes present in a sample, there are two types of analysis, namely **quantitative** and **qualitative**. Both types of test are employed to look for changes in a polyclonal distribution of antibody or to investigate the type of paraprotein found by electrophoresis.

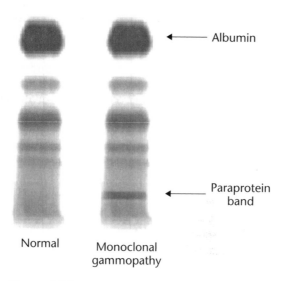

Figure 15.2
An electrophoresis strip showing a paraprotein band in the gamma region.

Quantitative measurements of each antibody class can indicate if a particular antibody is being made in excess, possibly due to a tumour, and indicate whether any of the antibody isotypes are being suppressed. A general increase in all isotypes may indicate a generalized immune response to an infection. Changes in antibody concentrations can be used as a measure of the effectiveness of therapy for monoclonal gammopathy.

If a paraprotein has been detected by electrophoresis, qualitative investigations are used to identify which particular antibody class is giving rise to the monoclonal antibody; this investigation is called antibody typing. The class of antibody present in the paraprotein can be important in determining the prognosis for the patient.

15.4   LABORATORY TECHNIQUES IN THE INVESTIGATION OF ANTIBODIES

The quantitative and qualitative investigations of antibodies present in serum and urine all employ specific antibodies raised in an animal that will react to a specific antibody isotype. This immune reaction is used in two different types of technique: one giving quantitative information – immunoprecipitation, and the other giving qualitative information – immunofixation.

Immunoprecipitation

Measurement of antibody isotypes can be carried out using anti-isotypic antibodies (an anti-IgG, for example) raised in a host animal such as a sheep or donkey. The anti-isotype antibody binds to the human protein, forming an insoluble immune complex that precipitates out of solution, called an **immunoprecipitate**. This reaction can be performed in a gel matrix, for example agarose gel, or in solution.

In gels, the anti-isotypic antibody is evenly distributed within the gel matrix. A couple of microlitres of sample are placed in a well cut into the gel. The sample is either allowed to diffuse though the gel or it is forced through the gel by electrophoresis. In the case where the sample diffuses through the gel, rings of immunoprecipitate are formed. The diameter of the ring is proportional to the concentration of human protein (antibody) being measured in the sample. This is called a **single radial diffusion technique** or sometimes, after its inventor, the **Mancini technique**. In the second case, where the sample is forced through the gel by electrophoresis, a rocket-shaped peak of immunoprecipitate is formed. The height of the peak is proportional to the concentration of the protein being measured in the sample. This technique is known as the **Laurell monorocket technique** after its inventor. Both these techniques give the same information, i.e. the concentration of protein in the sample. The Mancini technique takes approximately 48 hours before the results are ready, whilst Laurell monorockets require only a few hours. In practice the immunoprecipitate can be stained to make the measurement of the ring diameter or the peak height easier. *Figure 15.3* shows the types of result seen in these tests.

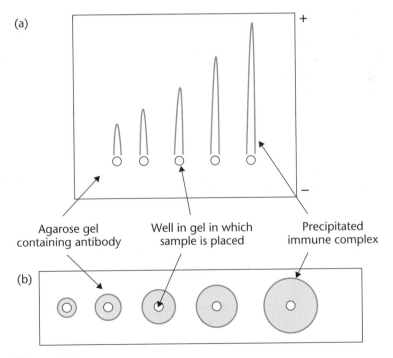

Figure 15.3
Immunoprecipitation in gel using (a) the Laurell monorocket technique, and (b) the radial immunodiffusion (Mancini) technique.

In the modern clinical biochemistry laboratory many immunoprecipitation reactions are performed on automated analysers, allowing the rapid analysis of many samples. In these methods the immunoprecipitate is formed in solution. Quantitation of the precipitate is by turbidometric (light absorption) or nephelometric (light scattering) readings. These tests take only a few minutes but are relatively expensive in terms of antibody usage. These methods are routinely used to measure levels of IgG, IgM and IgA in serum, urine and cerebrospinal fluid samples.

Immunofixation

Once a paraprotein has been demonstrated in a sample, the next stage in the investigation is to **type** the antibody that is giving the paraprotein. This is usually done by immunofixation, which employs agarose gel electrophoresis to separate the serum proteins into bands. The sample being investigated is run six times (in six different lanes, often with an empty lane between each) on the same electrophoresis plate. One run is stained with a total protein stain to give an overall pattern and to identify the position of the paraprotein on the electrophoresis strip. On each of the other lanes, where the sample has been run, the agarose gel is overlaid with a piece of filter paper, cut to the same size as the sample lane and soaked in a specific antibody. Five different antibodies are used: anti-IgG, anti-IgM, anti-IgA, anti-kappa light chain and anti-lambda light chain. The antibodies diffuse through the gel and form an immunoprecipitate with the separated human proteins in the sample. An antibody that reacts with the paraprotein will produce a discrete band of immunoprecipitate. The immunoprecipitate

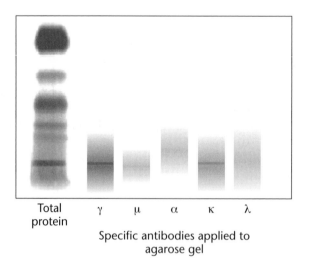

| Total protein | γ | μ | α | κ | λ |

Specific antibodies applied to
agarose gel

Figure 15.4
Results of an immunofixation to type a paraprotein. The specific antibodies react with heavy and light chains and form a band if they react with the paraprotein. In this case the patient has an IgG kappa paraprotein.

remaining in the gel is washed and stained and then the paraprotein is easy to type. A band of immunoprecipitate will appear in the same position as the band on the electrophoresis strip stained for total protein, for a given antibody. For example, a paraprotein will be typed as an IgG kappa if a band is seen in the lanes where anti-IgG and anti-kappa were applied.

Figure 15.4 shows the results from an immunofixation investigation showing the bands formed in particular lanes. Immunofixation is also used to identify Bence–Jones protein in urine samples.

SUGGESTED FURTHER READING

In addition to relevant chapters in the textbooks cited in Chapter 1 the following references are recommended.

Dispenzieri A. and Kyle R.A. (2005) Multiple myeloma: clinical features and indications for therapy. *Best Practice & Research Clinical Haematology*, **18**: 553–568.

Merlini G. (1995) Monoclonal gammopathies. *Cancer Journal*, **8**: 173–180.

San Miguela J.F., Gutiérreza N.C., Mateoa G. and Orfao A. (2006) Conventional diagnostics in multiple myeloma. *European Journal of Cancer*, **42**: 1510–1519.

Winearls C.G. (2003) Paraprotein-related renal disease and amyloid. *Medicine*, **31**: 99–100.

SELF-ASSESSMENT QUESTIONS

1. What are the five human antibody isotypes?
2. How many antigen-binding sites does IgM have?
3. Which cells synthesize antibody?
4. Which antibody isotype can cross the placenta?
5. Which antibodies can activate complement?
6. What is Bence–Jones protein?
7. What is the immunoglobulin being produced in abnormal amounts in macroglobulinaemia?
8. What name is given to a monoclonal antibody identified on an electrophoresis strip?
9. Which technique relies on the formation of different sized rings of immunoprecipitate to measure human antibody concentrations?

Proteins of the innate immune system

> **Learning objectives**
> *After studying this chapter you should confidently be able to:*
>
> ■ **Describe the innate immune system.**
> The innate immune system is non-specific and comprises the skin (physical barrier), phagocytic cells and soluble proteins. The most important proteins form complement, which is a group of proteins that act together to destroy bacteria and other foreign cells.
>
> ■ **Outline the activation pathways of complement.**
> Complement has two activation pathways. The classical pathway is activated by interaction with immune complexes and the alternative pathway is activated directly by some bacteria. Complement activation results in cell lysis via the membrane attack complex. C3b can act as an opsonin and C5a can act as a chemotactic factor, with C3a and C5a being anaphylatoxins.
>
> ■ **Give examples and roles of important acute-phase proteins.**
> Acute-phase protein synthesis is mediated by cytokines. Serum concentrations of acute-phase proteins increase during inflammation or injury. CRP is the most commonly measured acute-phase protein. Haptoglobin binds free haemoglobin. Alpha and beta interferons are anti-viral in their action.
>
> ■ **Outline investigation of proteins of the innate immune system.**
> CH_{50} is a measure of the whole classical complement activation pathway. Depletion of C3 and C4 indicates prolonged activation of the classical pathway. Depletion of C3 with normal C4 indicates prolonged activation of the alternative pathway.

In the previous chapter we saw how antibodies give protection against bacteria and viruses that can cause disease. The antibodies were produced as a response to a specific infective agent and the antibody bound to that particular infectious agent via specific interactions. In contrast to this acquired immunity, the innate immune system does not use specific interactions to give protection against infectious agents. The innate immune system does not require time to develop, it is ready for instantaneous action, it has no memory associated with it and it is not specific for any particular antigen. There are three principal components of the innate immune system:

- Physical barriers;
- Phagocytic cells;
- Soluble proteins.

The physical barriers include the skin and mucosal membranes lining the gut, lungs and urinary tract. These prevent the entry of bacteria and have bactericidal secretions on their surface, for example sweat. If damage occurs to the physical barriers, then phagocytic cells can engulf and digest bacteria; the principal phagocytic cell is the neutrophil. Some phagocytic cells such as monocytes can activate the acquired immune system. The most interesting of the three components to the clinical biochemist are the soluble proteins that protect the body from bacterial infection, prevent the spread of viral infection and aid the activation of the acquired immune system. The important proteins involved with the innate immune system are:

- Complement;
- Acute-phase proteins;
- Interferons.

In this chapter we will explore the biochemical facets of the innate immune system (see *Box 16.1*).

Box 16.1 Complement

In 1894 Richard Pfeiffer discovered that particular bacteria (cholera bacilli) were lysed when mixed with antiserum from a guinea pig that had been inoculated with that bacteria. He demonstrated that two components were required for lysis of the bacteria: antibodies and a heat-labile fraction of the antiserum. It was in 1895 that Charles Bordet confirmed that fresh serum was able to lyse bacteria at normal body temperature but if he heated the serum to 56°C the serum lost its ability to lyse the bacteria. He termed this heat-labile fraction 'alexine'. It was later that Ehrlich first used the term 'complement' to describe the component in plasma that helped antibodies cause bacterial lysis, displacing the term 'alexine'. The discovery of complement is usually ascribed to Bordet.

16.1 COMPLEMENT PROTEINS

Complement is a group of proteins which act together in order to destroy invading bacteria or other foreign cells. There are 20 or so complement proteins, some of which are complexed together to form 11 main proteins, and many of these are proenzymes, becoming active when one of the other complement proteins cleaves part of the molecule. This means that the complement system is a cascade of enzymes, each activating the next, resulting in an amplification effect. Many of the complement proteins form part of a complex which is built on the cell surface. The result is a pore-like structure inserted into the cell membrane: the membrane attack complex (MAC). This causes the lysis and destruction of the cell. During activation of the MAC, some of the complement proteins are cleaved, releasing a soluble component. These soluble fractions have a number of physiological actions which give rise to many of the symptoms seen in inflammation. Following cleavage, the soluble fraction has the suffix 'a' and the membrane-bound portion the suffix 'b'; for example, after cleavage C3 becomes C3a (soluble) and C3b (membrane-bound). The complement proteins have the letter C followed by a number. C1 is a complex of three proteins: C1q, C1r and C1s. The sequence of reactions is:

C1, C4, C2, C3, C5, C6, C7, C8, C9

There are two pathways of complement activation. The first is the **classical pathway** and this involves the sequential activation of the above complement proteins. The other pathway is known as the **alternative pathway** and is initiated by a number of factors called simply factors B and P. The important difference between these two pathways is the way in which they are activated. The classical pathway is activated by an immune complex interacting with C1. For this to take place the immune system must already be synthesizing antibody. In contrast, the alternative pathway can be activated directly by some bacteria.

During complement activation two important enzymes are formed by aggregation of surface-bound products. The first is C3 convertase, formed from the membrane-bound products of C4 and C2, and the second is C5 convertase, formed by adding C3b to C3 convertase. The activation of complement by the two pathways is shown in *Fig. 16.1*.

C3b serves another function on the surface of cells or bacteria, as it can enhance the action of the phagocytic cells, thereby promoting a more rapid destruction. This process is called **opsonization** and the C3b is acting as an **opsonin**.

Complement not only causes cell lysis but, during its activity, the release of the soluble component C5a causes the attraction of phagocytic cells to the area of activation; this is known as **chemotaxis**. C3a and C5a are **anaphylatoxins** and have potent physiological action, being able to cause mast cells to release histamine into the surrounding tissues, a process known as **anaphylaxis**.

16.2 ACUTE-PHASE PROTEINS

Following acute inflammation, as seen during infections, after surgery or sometimes in the presence of tumours, a number of serum proteins have increased concentration. In some cases the increase can be as much as 1000-fold. These proteins are known as acute-phase proteins or acute-phase reactants. The liver is the site of synthesis for most of these proteins. The production of these acute-phase proteins is controlled by a number of **cytokines** – chemical messengers released by cells of the innate immune system during an inflammatory response (see *Box 16.2*). The more important cytokines are:

■ Tumour necrosis factor;
■ Interleukin-1 (IL-1);
■ Interleukin-6 (IL-6).

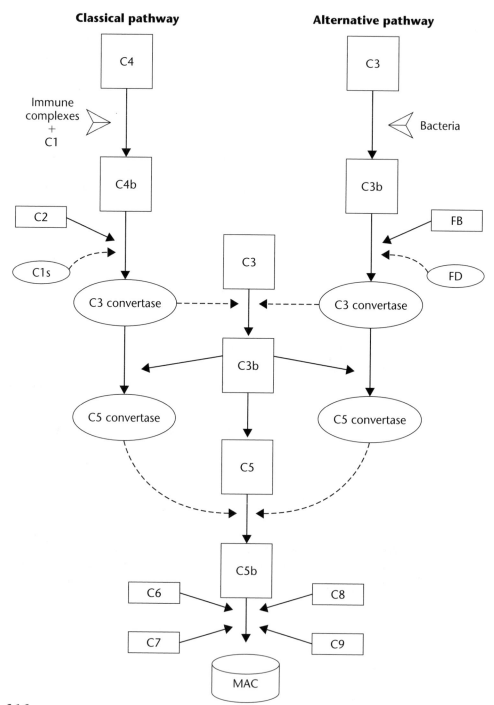

Figure 16.1
The activation of complement by the classical and alternative pathways. The activation points of the two pathways are shown by arrowheads. Square boxes show complement proteins that are cleaved or become part of a larger complex; elliptical boxes show those enzymatically active complement proteins or complexes; and the dashed lines show the site of enzymatic action. FB = factor B; FD = factor D; MAC = membrane attack complex.

Box 16.2 Cytokines

Cytokines are chemicals, released from cells, that regulate the growth and differentiation of other cells. They are often low molecular weight glycoproteins secreted in nanomolar amounts. Interleukin is the term used for cytokines that act among populations of leukocytes, and lymphokines are cytokines derived from lymphocytes. In 1994, 50 cytokines were recognized and now over 150 cytokines have been identified.

Table 16.1 lists the more important acute-phase proteins measured in the clinical biochemistry laboratory and gives an indication of the degree of elevation above the reference range that might be seen. Further information is given below on three of the acute-phase proteins most likely to be encountered in the less specialized clinical biochemistry laboratory.

Table 16.1 Acute-phase proteins classified according to the degree of elevation above the reference range that might be seen during an acute-phase response

Up to a 1000-fold increase in concentration:
> C-reactive protein; serum amyloid A

2- to 4-fold increase in concentration:
> α_1-Antichymotrypsin; α_1-antitrypsin; α_1-acid glycoprotein; fibrinogen; haptoglobin

1.5-fold increase in concentration:
> Ceruloplasmin; C3 and C4

C-reactive protein

By far the most commonly measured acute-phase protein is C-reactive protein (CRP), described in Chapter 12. Its major role is to bind to certain bacteria, acting as an opsonin, and enhance phagocytosis of the bacteria. It is commonly used to screen for acute inflammation and to monitor the progress of inflammatory conditions such as rheumatoid arthritis. Another common use is for screening children for bacterial infections (see *Box 16.3*).

Haptoglobin

Haptoglobin is a group of proteins, synthesized within the liver, adipose tissue and the lung. Their function is to remove free haemoglobin that has been released into the tissue fluids and blood in cases of haemolysis, as free haemoglobin can be toxic. They transport the haemoglobin to the reticulo-endothelial system where the iron is recovered. As haptoglobin is utilized in this process, in cases where there is extensive haemolysis, serum levels of

---

Box 16.3 Inflammation

The signs of inflammation were first described in the first century AD by the Roman physician Cornelius Celsus. These are:

Rubor	(redness)
Calor	(heat)
Tumor	(swelling)
Dolor	(pain)

These symptoms are mediated by proteins released from cells, or by activated plasma proteins, in response to inflammation. Important proteins include histamine, cytokines and complement proteins, many being acute-phase proteins. Redness and heat are caused by vasodilation. Swelling is caused by local vascular permeability and oedema. Pain is enhanced by the action of some of the activated proteins on pain receptors and by the stretching of tissue due to swelling.

---

haptoglobin are reduced. In the acute-phase response, levels of haptoglobin increase (and hence it is an acute-phase protein), but this increase may be masked by increased utilization due to haemolysis. It is for this reason that haptoglobin levels should be interpreted in conjunction with other acute-phase proteins such as CRP.

α_1-Antitrypsin

α_1-Antitrypsin is a protease inhibitor, especially of elastase and proteases released by leukocytes. It is synthesized within the liver and increases in concentration during an acute-phase reaction. α_1-Antitrypsin deficiency is associated with the destruction of tissue where there is a high content of elastase and collagen, for example the lungs. This deficiency can be due to protein-losing states or due to an inborn error of metabolism (affecting young children) where an abnormal protein is made which cannot be secreted. This can accumulate in the liver, leading to cirrhosis. The patient also has pulmonary emphysema.

16.3 INTERFERONS

The innate immune system is aided by two cytokines, called alpha interferon (IFN-α) and beta interferon (IFN-β). There is also a gamma interferon but this is concerned with controlling the cellular response of the acquired immune system. IFN-α and IFN-β are released by cells of the innate immune system in response to infection or injury. Their major function is to inhibit viral replication, preventing the spread of viral infection, and to inhibit cell proliferation. Analysis of interferons is a specialist investigation and is not performed routinely.

16.4 CLINICAL BIOCHEMISTRY AND THE INNATE IMMUNE SYSTEM

Investigation in the clinical biochemistry laboratory involves measurement of the proteins of the innate immune system. Many of these assays are specialized investigations and would only be performed in a specialist centre. However, the measurement of CRP is widely performed and in some A&E departments this is a 'near-patient' test.

Complement investigations

These days complement proteins are measured using an immunoassay but not so many years ago complement activity was measured by its ability to lyse red blood cells. This was a functional assay giving an overview of the whole of the complement pathway. It was known as the CH_{50} test and measured the ability of complement to induce lysis of sheep red blood cells (SRBCs) which had been coated with antibody. In the test the patient's serum was diluted 1 in 50 and then serially diluted, giving a range of dilutions. Each dilution was incubated with the SRBCs and the complement proteins in the patient's serum would lyse the red cells, each dilution giving less haemolysis as the complement proteins became more dilute. The dilution that gave 50% haemolysis was called the CH_{50}. The greater the amount of complement present in the sample, the greater the dilution needed to haemolyse 50% of the SRBCs.

The CH_{50} is decreased if one or more of the complement proteins are present in decreased concentrations. If one of the complement components is absent there will be no lysis and the CH_{50} is recorded as zero.

The CH_{50} test is reliant on antibody-coated red blood cells and it is only the classical pathway that is being tested. Modern methods measure individual complement proteins, relying on specific antibodies in an immuno-type assay. Often immunoprecipitation techniques (see Chapter 15) are used for the complement protein estimations. Listed below are the more common complement proteins that are measured and their reference ranges.

C1q	0.11–0.21 g l^{-1}
C3	0.8–1.8 g l^{-1}
C4	0.15–0.5 g l^{-1}
C5	0.07–0.17 g l^{-1}

Increased levels of C3, C4 and CH_{50} are seen in response to inflammation, as the complement proteins are also acute-phase reactants. Increased levels are seen primarily in autoimmune disease, infections and other trauma such as acute myocardial infarction.

Low levels of complement or a low CH_{50} indicate one of the following:

■ Increased consumption of complement proteins;
■ Decreased synthesis of complement proteins;
■ The presence of a complement inhibitor;
■ A congenital deficiency of one or more complement proteins.

Prolonged activation of complement will lead to the consumption of complement proteins, and measurement of specific complement proteins will give an indication of which pathway has been activated. The more important assays are those for C3 and C4. If the classical pathway has been activated a depletion of C4 and C3 is seen, indicating that antibody–antigen complexes are involved. This could be due to an infection or an auto-immune disease, where the body makes antibody against itself, forming immune complexes. Much of the damage seen in autoimmune disease comes from complement activation and the destruction of the tissue to which the antibody binds.

Depletion of C3 but not C4 indicates activation of the alternative pathway due predominantly to bacterial infection.

Acute-phase proteins and interferons

Measurement of these proteins is by immunoassay and there are a wide variety of methods in use, ranging from enzyme immunoassays to rapid screening tests using the agglutination of latex particles coated with antibody to the acute-phase protein. This latter technique is employed in the rapid determination of CRP.

SUGGESTED FURTHER READING

Kaufmann S. (2004) *Innate Immune System*. Washington, DC: American Society for Microbiology.

Ley K. (ed.) (2000) *Physiology of Inflammation*. New York: Oxford University Press.

Morgan B.P., Marchbank K.J., Longhi M.P., Harris C.L. and Gallimore A.M. (2005) Complement: central to innate immunity and bridging to adaptive responses. *Immunology Letters*, **97**: 171–179.

Szebeni J. (ed.) (2004) *The Complement System: Novel Roles in Health and Disease*. New York: Kluwer Academic Publishers.

Wen L., Atkinson J.P. and Giclas P.C. (2004) Clinical and laboratory evaluation of complement deficiency. *Journal of Allergy and Clinical Immunology*, **113**: 585–593.

SELF-ASSESSMENT QUESTIONS

1.   What are the two activation pathways of complement?
2.   What is the process called where a bacterium is coated with a molecule to aid phagocytosis?
3.   What is the name of the group of proteins that cause cell lysis following complement activation?
4.   Which compounds initiate the release of acute-phase proteins?
5.   Which acute-phase proteins can show a 1000-fold increase in concentration?

6. What is the function of haptoglobin?
7. Which proteins of the innate immune system have antiviral properties?
8. If no functional complement was found in a sample, what would the CH_{50} be?
9. Depletion of C3 but not C4 suggests activation of which complement pathway?

Kidney function

Learning objectives
After studying this chapter you should confidently be able to:

■ **Explain normal kidney function.**
The functional unit of the kidney is the nephron. The kidney removes waste products, reabsorbs essential compounds and regulates water, electrolyte and acid–base homeostasis. The kidney produces two hormones, 1,25-dihydroxycholecalciferol and erythropoietin. The glomerulus filters blood producing glomerular filtrate. The glomerular filtration rate is how much glomerular filtrate is produced in 1 minute.

■ **Classify the main types of kidney disease.**
Loss of kidney function can be classified by the cause; pre-renal conditions, renal disease or post-renal pathology. Acute renal failure often resolves. Chronic renal failure is irreversible. Oligouria is a low urine volume (<400 ml day^{-1}) and anuria is no urine production.

■ **Describe the common biochemical tests of kidney function.**
Blood concentrations of urea and creatinine are indicators of renal disease. Glomerular function can be assessed by measuring creatinine clearance. Tubular function can be assessed by measuring the urinary concentration of compounds normally absorbed or excreted by the kidney, e.g. amino acids or hydrogen ions.

■ **Describe the diagnostic role of urinary proteins.**
Proteinuria is an abnormal amount of protein in the urine (>150 mg day^{-1}). Analysis of urinary proteins can help to differentiate between glomerular and tubular disease. Microalbuminuria is an abnormal elevation of urinary albumin concentration above normal but below the detection limit of a urine dip-stick test for albumin.

In this section of the book we will study **output** from the body by looking at two major organs – the kidney and the liver. We have seen that in order to maintain health we need to:

■ **Input** nutrients;
■ **Control** and regulate the function of organs in the body;
■ **Process** nutrients to build cells and produce energy for life;
■ **Transport** various molecules around the body in order that processing may take place;

- Have a **defence** mechanism to give protection against pathogenic material;
- **Output** or remove waste products from the body to prevent the build-up of toxic products.

As we have seen, if any of these processes becomes damaged or malfunctions the result is a pathological process resulting in clinical symptoms. Some may be only trivial, whereas other may be life-threatening.

In this chapter we will consider the kidney, an organ with a major role in the removal of waste products, and in the final chapter we will study the liver, which is sometimes overlooked as an excretory organ. To be complete, we should mention the lungs and the gut as excretory organs. We have considered lungs and associated diseases in Chapter 14 and the gut in Chapter 3. The liver is part of the excretory system involving the gut and, as mentioned, is studied in the next chapter.

The kidneys are important organs essential for life. There are two kidneys each weighing approximately 150 g and measuring approximately 12 cm in length. They filter the blood and regulate its **biochemical composition**, and hence the kidneys are important organs in the investigation of biochemical abnormalities. The role of the kidneys is to:

- Remove water-soluble waste products from the blood;
- Regulate water, electrolyte and acid–base balance;
- Reabsorb essential compounds.

Waste products are formed as an end product of protein and nucleic acid metabolism, resulting in the production of urea, creatinine, creatine and uric acid. The end products of carbohydrate metabolism are energy, carbon dioxide (removed by the lungs) and water. Lipid metabolism creates lipid-soluble waste products that are excreted by the liver. The kidneys regulate water and electrolyte balance (see Chapter 7) and acid–base balance (see Chapter 14), and also respond to hormones that regulate calcium and phosphate balance (Chapter 8). Besides being a target organ for a number of hormones, the kidney is also an endocrine organ producing hormones, the important ones being:

- 1,25-Dihydroxycholecalciferol, which acts on the gut, promoting calcium absorption;
- Erythropoietin, which acts on the bone marrow, promoting haemoglobin synthesis.

The kidney acts as a salvage organ, recovering material from the filtered blood such as glucose and amino acids (see *Box 17.1*).

17.1 KIDNEY STRUCTURE AND FUNCTION

The kidney contains many millions of **nephrons** that act by filtering the blood and producing urine. The nephron, shown in *Fig. 17.1*, can be divided into the **glomerulus**, **proximal tubule**, **loop of Henle** and the **distal tubule**,

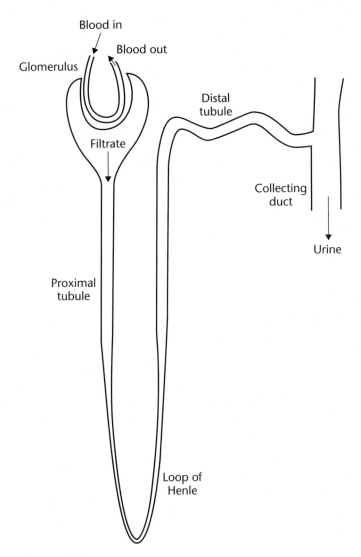

Figure 17.1
Diagram of a nephron.

that drains into a **collecting duct**. These different areas of the nephron have different functions associated with them.

Glomerulus

This is a 'funnel' of cells, making up the **Bowman's capsule**, in which a 'knot' of capillaries is found. Fluid in the blood is filtered through the glomerular basement membrane, leaving behind blood cells and large molecules such as proteins. The basement membrane can be thought of as having pores, through which small molecules pass. In reality the filtering mechanism is more complex. Small proteins pass through the membrane into the filtrate, and the larger the protein, the smaller the percentage that passes into the filtrate. For example, albumin has a plasma concentration of 35–50 g l^{-1}, but in the glomerular filtrate the concentration is 100–300 mg l^{-1}.

The kidney filters 1200 ml of blood per minute, which produces 120 ml of filtrate. The exact amount depends on a number of factors including the renal blood flow and pressure, the integrity of the glomerular basement membrane and the number of functioning nephrons.

An important measure of glomerular function is the **glomerular filtration rate** (GFR), which is how much filtrate is produced in a given time. The normal GFR is approximately 130 ml min^{-1} for a young adult male. The GFR is related to the size of the individual, so that a calculated GFR has to be adjusted according to the approximate surface area of the individual (calculated from height and weight). The normal GFR is:

$$130 \text{ ml min}^{-1} \text{ } 1.73 \text{ m}^{-2}$$

The GFR drops by approximately 10% per decade after the age of 35 due to loss of functional nephrons.

Proximal tubule

The glomerular filtrate passes into the proximal tubule (also called the proximal convoluted tubule) where most of the essential compounds filtered at the glomerulus are reabsorbed. For most compounds this is an active reabsorption, each compound having its specific reabsorption mechanism. Water, on the other hand, is passively reabsorbed along with sodium ions, which are absorbed via a sodium pump. *Table 17.1* shows the amounts filtered at the glomerulus compared with amounts lost in the urine for some compounds. Glucose in the glomerular filtrate is fully reabsorbed and in health does not appear in the urine. If the concentration in the blood and hence the concentration in the glomerular filtrate exceeds 10 mmol l^{-1}, the absorption mechanism is saturated and the excess glucose appears in the urine. The proximal tubule is also the site of protein reabsorption, where 95% is recovered.

Loop of Henle

The loop of Henle has a descending limb and an ascending limb found in the medulla of the kidney. This is the site of sodium and chloride reabsorption, which is brought about by osmotic mechanisms called **countercurrent multiplication** and **countercurrent exchange**.

Table 17.1 Comparison of the amounts of certain substances in the glomerular filtrate and the amounts excreted in the urine

	Amount filtered (mmol day^{-1})	Amount excreted in urine (mmol day^{-1})
Sodium	25 000	100
Bicarbonate	4500	<5
Urea	900	600
Potassium	600	50
Calcium	200	7.5
Phosphate	200	25
Magnesium	100	5
Uric acid	45	6
Creatinine	18	20
Water (litres day^{-1})	180	1.5

Distal tubule

Also called the convoluted distal tubule, this is an important site for sodium, potassium and hydrogen ion regulation. Sodium is reabsorbed through specific ion channels under the control of the hormone aldosterone. As sodium is reabsorbed, potassium and hydrogen ions are lost. This is the major site of hydrogen ion excretion and bicarbonate reabsorption, as described in Chapter 14. Other hormones act on the cells of the distal tubule: antidiuretic hormone (ADH) enables the reabsorption of water and parathyroid hormone stimulates the reabsorption of calcium.

Collecting ducts

The collecting ducts have a similar role to that of the proximal tubule and are the site of the fine control of sodium and potassium balance. The major role of the collecting ducts is the reabsorption of more water, again under the influence of ADH. When little ADH is present the urine will be dilute and, conversely, if there are higher levels of ADH acting on the cells of the collecting duct then the urine produced is more concentrated.

17.2 KIDNEY DISEASE

For normal kidney function the following are required:

■ Adequate blood supply to the kidney;
■ Normal functioning kidney tissue;
■ Patent tubules, collecting ducts and urinary tract.

Diseases which disturb any of the above can lead to kidney damage and kidney failure. Diseases causing kidney damage can also be classified using the above criteria. This classification is shown below:

■ Pre-renal: loss of blood supply;
■ Renal: loss of functional kidney tissue;
■ Post-renal: blockage of urinary tract preventing urine outflow.

Table 17.2 gives an overview of different types of kidney disease, giving some examples. This chapter is devoted mainly to **renal disease**, i.e. diseases arising from the loss of functioning tissue. Damage can be brought about by infections, trauma, toxicity, tumours, immune damage and ischaemia, leading to necrosis.

Table 17.2 Examples of different types of disease resulting in loss of kidney function

Pre-renal:	Decrease in plasma volume
	Reduced cardiac output
	Occlusion of renal artery
Renal:	Acute
	Acute glomerulonephritis
	Tubular necrosis
	Nephrotoxicity, e.g. heavy metals, deposition of protein
	Septic shock
	Infections
	Chronic
	Glomerulonephritis
	Polycystic kidney disease
	Diabetic nephropathy
	Chronic pyelonephritis
Post-renal:	Renal stones
	Cancer of prostate

Kidney damage can be acute or chronic. In **acute renal failure** there is a sudden increase in plasma urea and creatinine over a few days. Acute renal failure is usually accompanied by **oligouria** (low urine volume <400 ml day^{-1}), or even **anuria** (no urine production), if there is an obstruction. This is followed by a period of diuresis where the urine volume increases. The patient often recovers normal kidney function. **Chronic renal failure**, on the other hand, shows a gradual increase in urea and creatinine over a period of weeks or months. In this type of disease there is destruction of kidney tissue that is irreversible, leading to end-stage renal failure.

Disease of the kidney often manifests itself with symptoms relating to biochemical changes that can be detected in the blood. From the above discussion we can see that kidney disease can result in one or more of the following:

- Accumulation of waste products, e.g. urea, creatinine;
- Unwanted loss of large molecules, e.g. proteins;
- Disordered water balance;
- Disordered electrolyte balance, e.g. sodium and potassium;
- Disordered acid–base balance;
- Disordered calcium balance;
- Anaemia.

When investigating kidney disease there may be a number of biochemical abnormalities present in the patient. Changes in sodium, potassium, calcium and acid–base balance are seen. More specific biochemical indicators of renal disease are markers of renal function and relate to how well the kidney is excreting waste products. The two important measures of renal function used in the clinical biochemistry laboratory are the urea and creatinine concentrations.

Urea is the end product of amino acid metabolism, formed from the breakdown of protein (reference range 3.3–6.7 mmol l^{-1}), and 100 g of protein produces approximately 30 g of urea. It is very water soluble and is freely filtered by the glomerulus and passes into the kidney tubules. In the collecting ducts, some urea is reabsorbed, the amount depending on the flow rate of the glomerular filtrate. About 40% is reabsorbed with high flow rates (>2.0 ml min^{-1}), but up to 60% is reabsorbed when the flow rate is low (0.5 ml min^{-1}).

Creatinine is derived from phosphocreatine found in muscle. Between 10 and 20 mmol of creatinine is produced each day. Creatinine is filtered by the glomerulus and passes through the nephron without reabsorption taking place. A small amount may be excreted into the urine via kidney tubule cells as indicated in *Table 17.1*. The reference range is age- and sex-related, reflecting the average muscle mass found in the reference population when divided into age groups and gender.

It is useful to consider two aspects of kidney function, namely:

- Glomerular function;
- Tubular function.

Glomerular function relates to the filtration of the blood and tubular function relates to aspects of reabsorption and secretion by the tubules.

17.3 GLOMERULAR FUNCTION

Glomerular function can be assessed by estimating the glomerular filtration rate (GFR) and also by studying the range of proteins let through by the glomerular basement membrane. In a clinical biochemistry laboratory a very crude assessment of the GFR can be made from the blood concentration of urea or creatinine. Urea passes through the glomerulus and, depending on the GFR, some is reabsorbed in the kidney tubules. As we have seen above, the slower the GFR, the more urea is reabsorbed, leading to an elevated plasma urea concentration. This is only a very crude reflection of

GFR as levels of urea are also influenced by the rate of urea production, and a high protein intake can lead to an elevated urea concentration. On the other hand, a low protein intake can result in a low plasma urea concentration, which could lead to renal insufficiency not being detected. A more accurate measure of GFR can be made using creatinine. Creatinine is filtered by the glomerulus and is not reabsorbed in the kidney tubule. The rate of excretion is related to the GFR only. In situations where the GFR is reduced, creatinine levels increase in the plasma as the creatinine cannot be excreted by the kidney efficiently. Although the creatinine concentration can reflect the GFR, creatinine itself is not an accurate measure of GFR. Other factors can affect the plasma creatinine concentration. Creatinine levels in the blood depend on the muscle mass of the patient, and diet can also influence levels, especially when large amounts of roasted meats have been eaten. Another factor is that, as the GFR decreases, some creatinine is secreted by the proximal tubules. Despite these limitations, creatinine is a simple and reasonably reliable indicator of GFR.

A more precise measurement of GFR is to determine the **clearance** of a substance filtered by the glomerulus. This is the volume of blood that is theoretically completely cleared of a substance in a given time. The formula for clearance is:

$$\text{Clearance} = \frac{UV}{P} \ (\text{ml min}^{-1})$$

where: U = the urinary concentration of the given substance (in mmol l^{-1}); V = the volume of urine produced (in ml min^{-1}); and P = the plasma concentration of the given substance (in mmol l^{-1}). The unit of clearance is ml min^{-1}.

If a substance is filtered by the glomerulus and passes through the kidney tubules without reabsorption or secretion of that substance, the clearance will equal the GFR. Inulin is one such substance; an inulin clearance test will give an accurate measure of GFR. In the routine clinical laboratory the **creatinine clearance** gives a suitable measure of GFR. The GFR measured by a creatinine clearance test will give results slightly higher than those obtained from an inulin clearance test, due to the small amount of creatinine secreted by the renal tubule. This is only a problem if renal failure becomes severe and a large proportion of the excreted creatinine is derived from secretion by the kidney tubule. In order to measure the creatinine clearance, a timed urine sample is required. However, accurate urine volumes are sometimes difficult to obtain and there are a number of formulae that have been derived which estimate the creatinine clearance from the plasma concentration only (see *Box 17.2*).

Glomerular damage can also be assessed by studying the molecular weight of the proteins passing through the kidney and appearing in the urine. This is dealt with later in the chapter under 'Proteinuria'.

Recently a new marker for the early assessment of GFR, called **cystatin C**, has been proposed. Cystatin C is a low molecular weight protein (13.3 kDa), consisting of 120 amino acids. It is freely filtered in the glomerulus and completely reabsorbed in the proximal tubules. The serum concen-

---

Box 17.2 Creatine clearance calculations

A 41-year-old male with suspected kidney disease had a serum creatinine level of 172 μmol l⁻¹. A 24 hour urine collection was made, which had a volume of 1990 ml and a creatinine concentration of 6.8 mmol l⁻¹. The creatinine clearance is given by:

$$\text{Creatinine clearance} = \frac{UV}{P}$$

Here: U = 6.8 mmol l⁻¹; P = 0.172 mmol l⁻¹; V = 1990 / (24 x 60) = 1.38 ml min⁻¹.
Therefore:

$$\text{Creatinine clearance} = \frac{6.8 \times 1.38}{0.172} = 54.6 \text{ ml min}^{-1}$$

This is a low result; for a healthy adult male the creatinine clearance should be around 130 ml min⁻¹. Above 35 years of age the clearance drops by about 10% per decade.

---

tration of cystatin C has been shown to be increased in cases of reduced GFR and is thought to have a better diagnostic accuracy than serum creatinine measurements. Methods and kits are available for serum cystatin C, but it is still seen as a specialized test, although more laboratories are beginning to offer measurements.

17.4 TUBULAR FUNCTION

The glomerular filtrate produced from filtering blood passes through the kidney tubules, where reabsorption of useful substances and the secretion and excretion of waste substances take place. These processes depend on having functional tissue, and in tubular disease there is a reduction in the amount of functioning tissue. Unlike tests of glomerular function, where the GFR can be readily assessed, there are no simple tests of tubular function. Indirect tests measure the presence of substances appearing in the urine, which should under normal circumstances be reabsorbed by the kidney. These substances include glucose, proteins and amino acids. Other tests work on the principle of loading the plasma with a substance that is normally excreted by the tubule and measuring its concentration in the urine. An example of such a test is the acid load test, where ammonium chloride is given to the patient to check that the kidney tubules excrete acid efficiently. A defective ability to secrete hydrogen ions by the tubules can result in acidosis, in this case called **renal tubular acidosis**.

One of the simplest tests of renal function is to assess the concentrating ability of the kidney by measuring the urine volume and osmolality. In health, water from the glomerular filtrate is reabsorbed by the tubules and collecting ducts, producing concentrated urine. A number of conditions exist where water is not fully reabsorbed, resulting in an excess volume of urine being produced (**polyuria**). The most important causes of polyuria are:

■ Increased water ingestion;
■ Diabetes insipidus;
■ Increased osmotic load.

17.5 PROTEINURIA

Proteinuria is the abnormal presence of protein in the urine, in excess of 150 mg day^{-1}. At the glomerulus, blood is filtered, allowing small protein molecules to pass into the glomerular filtrate. The concentration of protein in the glomerular filtrate is between 100 and 300 mg l^{-1}. Most of the protein is reabsorbed by the renal tubules and the amount excreted in the urine is less than 150 mg day^{-1}. The proteins that appear in normal urine consist of those filtered proteins, **albumin** and **micro-globulins**, and proteins secreted by the renal tubules, **secretory IgA** and **Tamm–Horsfall protein**.

The appearance of protein in the urine gives rise to four different types of proteinuria, depending on the source of the protein. These are:

■ **Glomerular proteinuria** arising from glomerular disease;
■ **Tubular proteinuria** arising from tubular disease;
■ **Overflow proteinuria** arising from the overflow of high plasma concentrations of low molecular weight protein;
■ **Secretory proteinuria** arising from protein secreted by the kidney tubule.

Analysis of the range of molecular weights of the proteins found in urine from patients with renal disease can aid in the differentiation between glomerular and tubular disease. Damage to the glomerular basement membrane can result in larger proteins being allowed through into the glomerular filtrate in greater amounts, causing glomerular proteinuria. In this case, protein appears in the urine when the reabsorptive capacity of the tubules is exceeded. Where damage to the glomerulus is limited or slight, an excess of albumin is found in the urine (**albuminuria**) whereas if damage to the basement membrane is more serious, increasingly large proteins are filtered by the glomerulus. In this situation proteins such as the immunoglobulins appear in the urine (see *Box 17.3*).

In health, 95% of the filtered protein is reabsorbed. This includes the small proteins allowed through the glomerular basement membrane: microglobulins, insulin and parathyroid hormone. Tubular damage impairs the uptake of these proteins, resulting in tubular proteinuria. *Table 17.3* demonstrates the above points numerically. Notice in particular the difference in the pattern of proteins excreted in the urine in glomerular and

---

Box 17.3 Renal disease

Richard Bright (1789–1858) was a pioneer of modern clinical biochemistry. He recognized the link between renal disease and the appearance of albumin in the urine.

Table 17.3 Comparison of urine protein excretion for albumin and low molecular weight proteins (LMWP) in normal, glomerular disease and tubular disease states

	Normal		Glomerular damage		Tubular damage	
	Albumin	LMWP	Albumin	LMWP	Albumin	LMWP
Plasma concentration (mg l^{-1})	4000	4	4000	4	4000	4
Filtered load (mg day^{-1})	360	360	360 000	360	360	360
Reabsorbed	95	95	95	95	50	50

tubular disease. Glomerular disease has higher levels of protein, often exceeding 2 g day^{-1}, mainly albumin, whereas tubular proteinuria shows a moderate increase in urinary proteins, usually less than 2 g day^{-1}, and shows an increased proportion of low molecular weight proteins. In clinical laboratories, the assessment of low molecular weight proteinuria is usually performed by measuring a single, low molecular weight protein, often β_2-microglobulin.

In the assessment of glomerular proteinuria, a useful investigation is the determination of the **selectivity** of the protein clearance by the kidney. Selectivity is the ability of the kidney to retain high molecular weight proteins whilst only low molecular weight proteins appear in the urine. If severe damage to the glomerular basement membrane is present, selectivity is lost as more high molecular weight proteins are lost in the urine. Where there has been only minimal damage to the glomerular basement membrane selectivity is maintained. By measuring the ratio of small to large proteins a **selectivity index** can be calculated:

$$\text{Selectivity index} = \frac{\text{Concentration of a small protein}}{\text{Concentration of a large protein}}$$

Typical proteins used as a measure of smaller proteins include albumin (68 kDa) and transferrin (80 kDa). Examples of proteins used for the larger protein determination are IgM (900 kDa) and α_2-macroglobulin (820 kDa).

As the proteinuria becomes more unselective, the amount of high molecular weight protein found in the urine increases, and the selectivity index falls. This can have a bearing on treatment given to the patient, as selective proteinuria is more likely to respond to steroid therapy.

Overflow proteinuria (sometimes called pre-renal proteinuria) occurs when abnormally high levels of a low molecular weight protein are present in the blood. The protein is filtered at the glomerulus and the high concentration saturates the tubule reabsorption capacity of the tubule, resulting in the remaining protein in the glomerular filtrate being lost in the urine. Examples of proteins associated with this type of proteinuria and associated conditions are shown in *Table 17.4*.

Table 17.4 Examples of proteins linked with overflow proteinuria and the associated conditions

Protein	Molecular weight (kDa)	Example of associated disease
Haemoglobin	68	Intravascular haemolysis
Myoglobin	17	Crush injuries, rhabdomyolysis
Immunoglobulin light chains	25	Multiple myeloma

In the final class of proteinuria, secretory proteinuria (sometimes called post-renal proteinuria), there is an increased production of inflammatory proteins secreted into the urinary tract. These proteins include secretory IgA and mucoproteins. The amount of protein released in this type of protein-uria is low and not easily demonstrated.

Protein analysis

Protein analysis is performed using a number of different techniques. An overall picture can be obtained from electrophoresis of the urine sample. The concentration of protein is normally very low, so that special sensitive staining methods are required, for example gold or silver staining, or the sample must be preconcentrated before electrophoresis. This is a good test for Bence–Jones protein, found in patients with a monogammopathy (see Chapter 15). Specific proteins are measured using specific antibodies in an immuno-type technique involving a simple immunoprecipitation or a labelled technique such as enzyme-linked immunosorbent assay (ELISA).

Microalbuminuria

Microalbuminuria refers to a small increase in the concentration of albumin above the normal, not to the size of the molecule. The elevation in concentration is slight and below the level of detection for the normal 'dipstick' method (this is positive at levels >250 mg day^{-1}). The normal level of albumin found in urine is 2.5–25 mg day^{-1}. The presence of microalbuminuria is used as an early marker of kidney damage for patients with diabetes mellitus (see Chapter 9). If left untreated this could develop into chronic renal failure.

Nephrotic syndrome

Unlike microalbuminuria, nephrotic syndrome involves the loss of very large amounts of protein in the urine. There is glomerular damage allowing the loss of between 2 and 30 g day^{-1} of protein. The main protein lost is albumin but other proteins can be involved. This loss leads to hypoalbuminaemia, oedema and secondary hyperaldosteronism (see Chapter 7).

Urine analysis

Urine provides an easily collected biological fluid on which a number of rapid screening tests can be performed. Not only can the urine composition help in assessing kidney disease but urine analysis can also give information about the presence of other diseases. The routine analysis of urine should include noting the appearance of the urine, the volume produced in a given time period, microbiological investigation and biochemical investigation. Biochemical investigation can fall into two types, namely screening and further investigation of renal disease.

Screening involves the use of simple chemical tests on a '**dipstick**'. These dipsticks have a number of impregnated pads attached to a plastic backing (the stick). Each pad contains the dried reagents required for the particular test. When the stick is dipped into a urine sample, the reagents are rehydrated and react with the urinary components. *Table 17.5* shows some of the more common urine dipstick tests available and examples of the diseases which would give an abnormal test result if the analyte appears in the urine in abnormally elevated amounts. The chemistry within the pad gives a coloured product and, generally, the more intense the colour, the more analyte present in the urine. The colour is compared against a standardized chart, allowing an approximation of the concentration of analyte to be made. This is a **semi-quantitative** measurement.

Table 17.5 Common urinary analytes measured using a 'dipstick' chemistry and examples of diseases which can cause an abnormal result

Analyte	Disease
Glucose	Diabetes
pH	Acidosis, renal disease
Albumin	Renal disease
Ketones	Diabetes
Bilirubin	Liver disease

New technology has enabled immune detection techniques to be incorporated into dipstick-type test strips, allowing rapid immunoassays to be used in urine screening. Examples of such tests include the detection of specific urine infections and drugs of abuse in police work.

Further investigation of renal disease uses conventional methodology on urine as well as blood samples. Such investigations include the measurement of urinary osmolality, sodium, potassium, hydrogen ions, calcium, creatinine and phosphate.

17.6   RENAL STONES

A small number of individuals (1 per 1000 males and 1 per 3000 females) will develop a renal stone (called a **calculus**), which may result in renal damage. The process of forming a kidney stone is **nephrolithiasis**. The formation of the stone is dependent on a number of factors including the presence of other pathology in the body, the concentration of the stone-forming material and the amount excreted, urinary volume, urinary flow, urinary pH and the presence of a urinary infection. The calculus consists of material that has come out of solution and has precipitated within the kidney. A 'seeding' process takes place, perhaps due to the presence of bacteria, in which layers of stone-forming material are deposited, gradually getting larger and larger. Calculi can be of many different shapes and sizes, ranging from the size of a grain of sand to stones several centimetres in diameter. There may be only one calculus or many hundreds of small calculi. Stones are analysed to ascertain their composition and the different types of material found in different stones are shown below. The list is in order of decreasing frequency.

- Calcium oxalate
- Calcium phosphate
- Magnesium ammonium phosphate
- Uric acid
- Cystine
- Xanthine

The analysis of renal calculi is traditionally performed using simple chemical analysis for calcium, oxalate, phosphate, etc. in test tubes. In more specialist laboratories where there is an interest in renal calculi, the analysis is performed using **infrared spectroscopy**. The infrared spectrum can identify the components of the renal calculi.

SUGGESTED FURTHER READING

In addition to relevant chapters in the text books cited in Chapter 1 the following references are recommended.

Beetham R. and Cattell W.R. (1993) Proteinuria – pathophysiology, significance and recommendations. *Annals of Clinical Biochemistry*, **30**: 425–434.

Christian M.T. and Watson A.R. (2004) The investigation of proteinuria. *Current Paediatrics*, **14**: 547–555.

Lameire N., Adam A., Becker C.R., *et al.* and CIN Consensus Working Panel (2006) Baseline renal function screening. *American Journal of Cardiology*, **98** (Supplement 1): 21–26.

Moutona R. and Holder K. (2006) Laboratory tests of renal function. *Anaesthesia and Intensive Care Medicine*, **7**: 240–243.

Rennke H.G., Denker B.M. and Rose B.D. (2006) *Renal Pathophysiology: the Essentials*, 2nd edition. Philadelphia: Lippincott Williams & Wilkins.

Samuell C.T. and Kasidas G.P. (1995) Biochemical investigations in renal stone formers. *Annals of Clinical Biochemistry*, **32**: 112–122.

Tencer J., Bakoush O. and Torffvit O. (2000) Diagnostic and prognostic significance of proteinuria selectivity index in glomerular diseases. *Clinica Chimica Acta*, **297**: 73–83.

SELF-ASSESSMENT QUESTIONS

1. Which two important hormones are synthesized in the kidney?
2. Where in the kidney is the blood filtered?
3. Where is the site of aldosterone action?
4. Will a high blood ADH produce a dilute or a concentrated urine?
5. Given a plasma creatinine concentration of 140 µmol l^{-1} and a 24 hour urine collection with a creatinine concentration of 15.2 mmol l^{-1} and a volume of 1650 ml, calculate the creatinine clearance.
6. What is the name given to an inability to secrete hydrogen ions from the kidney tubules?
7. How much protein is normally lost in the urine each day?
8. The severity of glomerular damage corresponds to which type of protein that appears in the urine in increasing amounts?
9. Which positive urine test would indicate liver disease?
10. How might a bacterium induce nephrolithiasis?

Liver function

Learning objectives
After studying this chapter you should confidently be able to:

- **Outline the structure and functions of the liver.**
  The liver is organized into lobules. Blood from the hepatic artery and portal vein passes across a large suface area of hepatocytes in the sinusoids. Heptocytes actively excrete bile into the bile canaliculi.

- **Describe the metabolism of bilirubin.**
  Bilirubin is formed from haem, mostly from decaying red blood cells. Bilirubin is not water soluble (but is lipid soluble) and is transported to the liver bound to albumin. Bilirubin is made water soluble by conjugating it with glucuronic acid. Conjugated bilirubin is excreted into the gut where it is converted to urobilinogen.

- **Outline different types of jaundice.**
  Jaundice is an elevated bilrubin concentration (hyperbilirubinaemia), which can classified according to the cause: pre-hepatic, hepatic and post-hepatic. Kernicterus is the deposition of bilirubin in lipid-rich brain tissue.

- **Broadly categorize different types of liver disease according to their biochemical profile.**
  Liver disease can be hepatocellular or cholestatic in origin. Hepatitis is the destruction of hepatocytes, releasing large amounts of intracellular enzymes, for example the transaminases. Cholestatis is the obstruction of the bile ducts and is associated with high levels of alkaline phosphatase. Alcoholic liver disease is characterized by increased levels of γ-glutamyl-transferase in the blood.

In the last chapter we saw how the kidneys removed water-soluble waste products in the urine. Lipid-soluble componds such as cholesterol and bilirubin cannot be excreted by this route. In this chapter we shall see how the liver is the route of excretion for many lipid-soluble compounds. It does this by metabolizing the lipid-soluble compound to form a water-soluble compound and then excretes it in the bile. In this chapter we shall study how the liver metabolizes bilirubin and consider how this metabolic pathway is disrupted in different liver diseases that result in high levels of bilirubin being found in the blood.

The liver is the major metabolic organ in the body and as such it has a number of important functions including:

- Metabolism of drugs;
- Synthesis of proteins;
- Metabolism of lipids;
- Carbohydrate metabolism;
- Storage of metabolic products;
- Excretion of lipid and bilirubin metabolites.

As you can see from the list above, the liver could be placed in the section concerned with processing or that dealing with transport and storage. However, because the investigation of liver disease in the clinical biochemistry laboratory is often centred on the level of bilirubin (a breakdown and waste product of haem) in the blood, this chapter on liver function is placed in the section concerned with output.

18.1   LIVER STRUCTURE

The liver weighs approximately 1500 g in the adult and has four lobes: the left, right, quadrate and caudate lobes. The liver lies just under the diaphragm on the right side. Blood enters the liver via the **hepatic artery** and via the **portal vein**, which carries blood from the gut, rich in absorbed nutrients. Leaving the liver is the hepatic vein and the left and right hepatic ducts, which carry bile to the gall bladder. Bile then drains into the gut where it is necessary in the digestion of lipid.

At the microscopic level, the liver is organized into **lobules**. The liver lobules are hexagonal in shape and contain a central vein from which radiate sheets of hepatocytes and some Kupffer cells (phagocytic cells of the reticulo-endothelial system that act as antigen-presenting cells). The space between these sheets of cells is called the sinusoid. Blood enters the sinusoids from the hepatic artery and the portal vein and drains into the central vein. A diagram of a liver lobule is shown in *Fig. 18.1*.

The sheets of hepatocytes are effectively one cell thick and have a very large surface area. The surfaces of the hepatocytes have many receptors for substances in the blood, allowing an efficient uptake of the relevant compounds from the blood into the hepatocytes. Examples of such receptors include LDL receptors, glycoprotein receptors and bilirubin receptors. Material from the blood on one side of the cells is 'picked up' and processed, and the hepatocytes release newly synthesized material or processed material either back into the blood (for example proteins or glucose) or into the bile on the other side of the cells (for example bilirubin and bile acids), which drains into the bile canaliculi and then into the hepatic ducts. A sheet of hepatocytes is illustrated in *Fig. 18.2*.

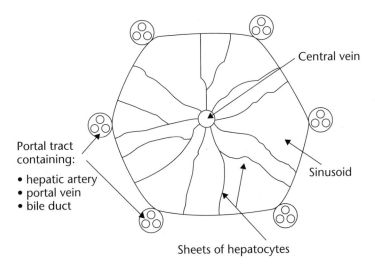

Figure 18.1
A liver lobule.

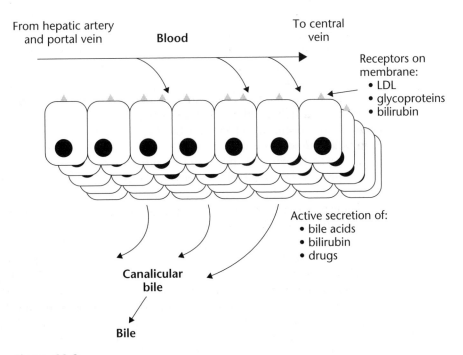

Figure 18.2
The flow of blood over sheets of hepatocytes that take up material from the blood via receptors on the cell surface. Lipid-soluble material such as bilirubin is conjugated and actively secreted into the bile.

18.2   BILIRUBIN METABOLISM

Bilirubin is a yellow compound, mostly formed from the breakdown of haemoglobin. Old or damaged red blood cells are broken down in the spleen, releasing **haemoglobin**. Haemoglobin is made from two pairs of protein chains, each carrying a **haem** group. Haem is a porphyrin ring holding an iron atom in the centre of the ring (see *Box 18.1*). Iron is recovered and the cyclic haem molecule is broken to form a linear compound called **biliverdin**. This is then reduced to give **bilirubin**. Approximately 35 mg of bilirubin is produced from 1 g of haemoglobin. About 80% of bilirubin formed is derived from the breakdown of old red blood cells, whilst the other 20% comes from the metabolism of immature blood cells and cytochromes.

Box 18.1 Structure of haemoglobin

The German organic chemist Hans Fischer was the first person to synthesize porphyrin molecules and showed that they were an important part of haemoglobin. He also discovered the structure of bilirubin and synthesized it in 1944.

Bilirubin is a lipophilic (lipid-soluble) molecule and is consequently insoluble in water. Albumin binds to bilirubin, acting as a transport protein, and carries it to the liver via the blood, entering the liver via the hepatic artery. The blood passes through the liver sinusoids, and in doing so it passes across the surface of the sheets of hepatocytes. Albumin carring bilirubin binds to specific receptors on the heptocyte surface and is taken into the cell. Bilirubin is removed from the albumin, which is recirculated.

In the hepatocyte, bilirubin is **conjugated** with **glucuronic acid** by the enzyme uridyl diphosphate glucuronosyltransferase (UDPGT). This conjugation results in a bilirubin molecule containing either one or two glucuronic acid residues, i.e. a mono- or diglucuronide. There is a greater proportion of monoglucuronide produced by the liver.

Conjugated bilirubin is water soluble and is actively secreted from the hepatocyte into the bile canaliculi, which eventually drain into the bile duct. The bile passes into the gut where bacteria reduce the conjugated bilirubin to **urobilinogen**. In the gut urobilinogen is sometimes called stercobilinogen. Most of the water-soluble urobilinogen is excreted in the faeces but some is absorbed by the gut and enters the blood stream, some is re-excreted by the liver (the enterohepatic circulation) and some is excreted in the urine. Urobilinogen is colourless but is oxidized to **urobilin** (or stercobilin), which is a brown-coloured compound. *Figure 18.3* shows the relationship between the structures of haem and conjugated and unconjugated bilirubin (see also *Box 18.2*).

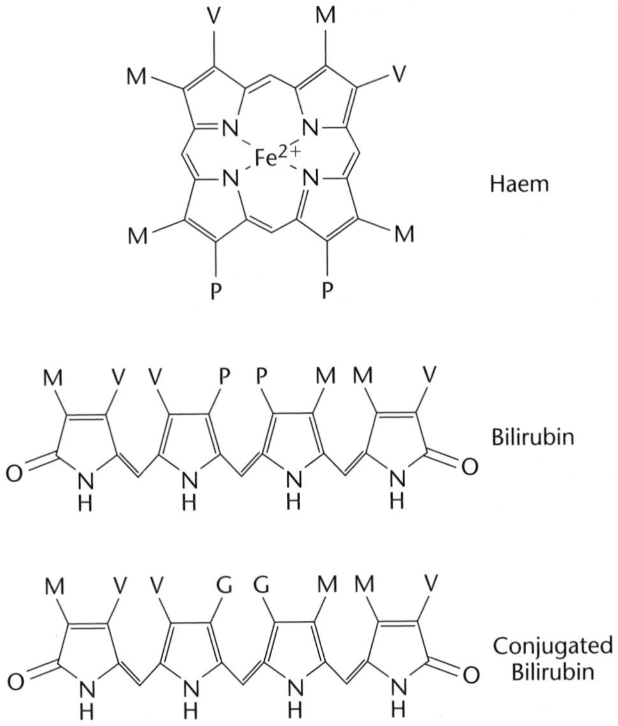

Haem

Bilirubin

Conjugated
Bilirubin

P = propyl ($-CH_2CH_2COOH$)
M = methyl ($-CH_3$)
V = vinyl ($-C= CH_2$)
G = glucuronic acid

Figure 18.3
Structures of haem and unconjugated and conjugated bilrubin.

Box 18.2 Bilirubin forms

Bilirubin can be fractionated by HPLC into four fractions:

- α fraction: unconjugated bilirubin; the major form in normal plasma, carried by albumin;
- β fraction: monoglucuronide bilirubin;
- γ fraction: diglucuronide bilirubin;
- δ fraction: a recently discovered fraction which is direct reacting (water soluble) and thought to be covalently bound to albumin.

18.3 JAUNDICE

Jaundice is the name given to a yellowish coloration found in patients with high levels of yellow pigment in their blood, and it is particularly apparent in the sclera of the eye. This is nearly always due to **hyperbilirubinaemia** (high blood bilirubin), although it can be seen where an excess of carrot juice has been taken (hypercarotenaemia), but this is very rare. The reference range for bilirubin is 0–18 µmol l^{-1} but jaundice does not become apparent until the blood level exceeds 40 µmol l^{-1}, and the yellow-looking plasma is said to be **icteric**.

Disruption of the bilrubin metabolic pathway (as previously described) by liver disease can lead to hyperbilirubinaemia and jaundice. In the remainder of this chapter, jaundice is equated with hyperbilirubinaemia.

Jaundice can be classified according to where the pathological lesion occurs, resulting in the three major groupings shown below.

■ Pre-hepatic jaundice: increased bilirubin synthesis;
■ Hepatic jaundice: hepatocellular disease and cholestatic disease;
■ Post-hepatic jaundice: biliary obstruction.

Figure 18.4 shows the relationship between the types of jaundice and the anatomical regions in which a disease process may give rise to a particular category of jaundice.

Pre-hepatic jaundice

This situation arises when an excessive amount of bilirubin is produced from an abnormally high breakdown of red cells, as may be seen in haemolytic anaemias or haemolytic disease of the newborn. In this type of jaundice, the bilirubin in the blood is unconjugated bilirubin; increased levels of conjugated bilirubin are formed and excreted in the bile, resulting in increased levels of urobilinogen being produced and, in turn, increased levels of urobilinogen are found in the urine. Unless there is any renal disease, no bilirubin is found in the urine.

Unconjugated bilirubin binds to albumin, but in cases of severe haemolytic disease of the newborn, for example due to a rhesus incompatibility, there may be so much bilirubin being produced that it saturates the available binding sites on albumin. If the blood level rises to more than 340 µmol l^{-1} (for full-term babies), the excess, free, unconjugated bilirubin, being lipid soluble, crosses the blood–brain barrier and dissolves in the lipid-rich brain tissue, staining the brain yellow. This is called **kernicterus**. Bilirubin is neurotoxic and kernicterus can result in brain damage to the baby.

Hepatic jaundice

In hepatic jaundice the hyperbilirubinaemia arises from disease processes within the liver and may thus involve hepatocellular disease and/or cholestatic disease. See the following section on liver disease for further details.

Post-hepatic jaundice

In conditions leading to post-hepatic jaundice there is a blockage of the bile duct, reducing or preventing bile flowing into the gut. This is mainly due

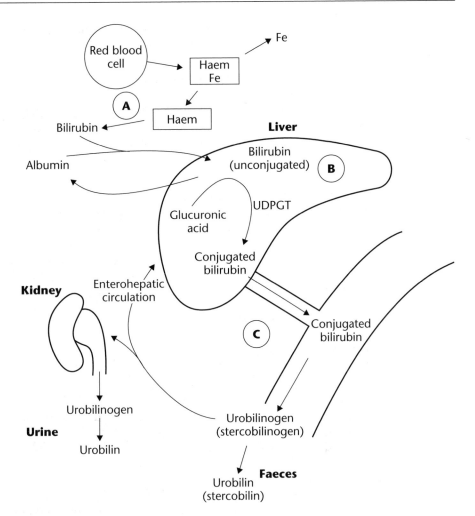

Figure 18.4
The metabolism of bilirubin. The letters represent areas where disease could result in jaundice; A – causes of pre-hepatic jaundice; B – causes of hepatic jaundice; C – causes of post-hepatic jaundice. UDPGT = uridyl diphosphate glucuronosyltransferase.

to the presence of gallstones or tumours, especially of the 'head' of the pancreas. The bile builds up a back pressure into the liver causing ruptur- ing of the bile canaliculi in the liver, and the bilirubin is forced back into the blood. The released bilirubin is conjugated and, being water soluble, it is freely filtered by the glomerulus and appears in the urine. If there is normal renal function, the presence of bilirubin in the urine is always a pathological finding. Because the bile duct is blocked the amount of biliru- bin reaching the gut is reduced and, consequently, less urobilinogen is formed, so that urinary bilinogen levels are reduced. A second consequence of reduced bile in the gut is that less urobilin (stercobilin) is formed, result- ing in pale-looking stools. Less fat is therefore absorbed as this requires bile acids (also found in the bile) and the stools are not only pale but also greasy or fatty.

Congenital hyperbilirubinaemia

There are four inborn errors of metabolism associated with bilirubin metabolism that result in hyperbilirubinaemia. Two of them give elevated levels of unconjugated bilirubin, whilst the other two give elevated levels of conjugated bilirubin. The four diseases are summarized below.

Gilbert's disease

This is a common condition that affects approximately 7% of the population. It is thought to be due to reduced activity of UDPGT, although a defective uptake mechanism may be involved. There is a slightly raised bilirubin, usually <50 μmol l^{-1}, which is unconjugated and, consequently, no bilirubin appears in the urine. This is an innocuous disease and many people may not even be aware that they are affected. The hyperbilirubinaemia becomes worse during times of stress due to infections or starvation.

Crigler–Najjar syndrome

Unlike Gilbert's disease this condition can be fatal. Here there is a lack of UDPGT activity, so that little or no bilirubin is conjugated, resulting in an unconjugated hyperbilirubinaemia. In the severe form there is a total deficiency of enzyme activity, leading to kernicterus and death of the newborn baby soon after birth. The milder form, where some enzyme activity is present, can be treated by drugs that can induce enzyme activity such as phenobarbitone.

Dubin–Johnson syndrome and Rotor syndrome

These rare conditions are caused by a defect in the excretion of bilirubin from the cell. This causes a conjugated hyperbilirubinaemia. Dubin–Johnson syndrome also involves porphyrin metabolism and the deposition of a black pigment in the liver.

18.4 LIVER DISEASE

Liver disease can be broadly divided into two categories according to the types of biochemical changes observed. These are **hepatocellular** conditions and **cholestatic** conditions. It must be borne in mind that one particular liver disease may show elements of both these categories.

Hepatocellular changes are seen with those diseases that result in damage to the hepatocytes. Cell damage can be caused by viral infections, and the effects of some drugs, chemicals and alcohol, leading to **hepatitis**. *Table 18.1* gives a short list of potential causes of hepatocellular damage. The resulting damage leads to changes in a wide range of biochemical parameters, some of which are measured in the clinical biochemistry laboratory and are used

Table 18.1 Some of the more common causes of liver disease classified according to the predominant biochemical changes observed

Hepatocellular changes		Cholestatic changes	
Viral:	Hepatitis A, B, C	*Intrahepatic obstruction:*	Acute hepatocellular damage
	Epstein–Barr virus		Structural liver damage
	Cytomegalovirus		Primary biliary cirrhosis
	Coxsackie virus		
Drugs:	Paracetamol		
	Isoniazid		
	Amoxycillin	*Extrahepatic obstruction:*	Gallstones
	Methotrexate		Pancreatitis
Chemicals:	Carbon tetrachloride		Malignancy
Toxins:	Aflatoxins		
	Alcohol		

to assess liver disease. The most important changes seen, from the point of view of routine investigations, are:

- Bilirubin levels increase, giving rise to jaundice; in hepatitis levels may reach 1000 μmol l^{-1}. Bilirubin in this instance is mainly conjugated.
- Hepatocyte damage releases enzymes from within the cell including the transaminases (see Chapter 10) and, as with bilirubin, very high levels are found in cases of hepatitis.
- In very severe cases of liver disease albumin levels (see Chapter 12) may be reduced as the liver has lost its synthesizing capability.

Cholestatic changes are seen as a result of **cholestasis**, which is an impairment in the flow of bile through the canaliculi and into the gut. A blockage can occur anywhere in the biliary tree and the causes of cholestasis can be conveniently categorized into **intrahepatic** and **extrahepatic** causes. *Table 18.1* shows some examples of conditions that result in cholestasis. A number of biochemical changes are associated with cholestasis and the main findings from routine investigations are:

- An elevated bilirubin, usually between 150 and 300 μmol l^{-1}, but gross elevation can sometimes be seen. The bilirubin will be predominantly conjugated.
- Elevated levels of alkaline phosphatase, as this enzyme is associated with the cells lining the bile canaliculi and bile ducts. Levels in excess of 1000 IU l^{-1} may be seen.
- The transaminases are usually normal or slightly elevated unless there is also hepatocellular damage, when higher levels may be found.

Some of the liver diseases investigated by the clinical biochemistry laboratory are described in more detail below.

Hepatitis

There are two types of hepatitis recognized, namely acute and chronic hepatitis. **Acute viral hepatitis** is due to viral destruction of the hepatocytes and can lead to dramatic changes in liver function test results. The disruption of the hepatocytes results in the loss of large amounts of intracellular enzymes into the blood and very high levels of transaminases are often recorded. Damage to hepatocytes also causes conjugated bilirubin to be lost in the blood, leading to elevated bilirubin levels. Acute hepatitis has three phases:

- Prodromal phase: fever, vomiting, abdominal pain and a general feeling of malaise. Jaundice is not evident at this stage but the urine may be dark in colour due to the presence of bilirubin. During this stage the transaminase levels are very high. Lasts 5–10 days.
- Icteric phase: jaundice is evident due to hyperbilirubinaemia. Lasts up to 3 weeks.
- Convalescent phase: abdominal pain and jaundice resolve and enzyme levels return to normal.

Viral infections resulting in hepatitis are from hepatitis A virus, associated with poor hygiene, hepatitis B virus and hepatitis C virus, both associated with infected blood or blood products. A number of other viral infections can result in viral hepatitis, in particular Epstein–Barr virus and cytomegalovirus.

Chronic hepatitis

Chronic hepatitis is defined as when there has been evidence of hepatic inflammation for longer than 6 months. This can follow acute hepatitis which fails to resolve, or it can be due to a chronic reaction to certain drugs or to an autoimmune disease.

Cirrhosis

Cirrhosis of the liver is a chronic progressive disease that leads to fibrosis of the liver (similar to scar tissue that develops after tissue damage). The biochemical picture shows cholestatic changes and a raised bilirubin, which is predominantly conjugated, but the level may be within the reference range during quiescent phases of the disease. Alkaline phosphatase is raised, often above 300 IU l^{-1}. Transaminases may be elevated, depending on the disease activity. As the disease progresses more active liver tissue is lost and the resulting loss of synthetic ability causes albumin levels in the blood to drop. In extreme cases they may fall to below 20 g l^{-1} and lead to ascites and oedema.

Alcoholic liver disease

The consumption of high levels of alcohol over long periods of time results in damage to the liver. A range of effects can be seen, depending on the extent of the damage and over what time the damage has accumulated. Minimal damage is reflected by an increase in the amount of liver enzymes in the blood, especially γ-glutamyltransferase (GGT). Further damage progressively leads to the development of 'fatty liver', alcoholic hepatitis and alcoholic cirrhosis. Cirrhosis develops as a result of hepatic tissue being replaced by fibrosis tissue, which occurs within 5–15 years of heavy alcohol abuse. Probably the most important biochemical finding in this condition is the elevated GGT, which is often disproportionately higher than the elevated alkaline phosphatase. This enzyme is often used as a marker of alcohol abuse, as up to 90% of heavy drinkers will have elevated GGT levels in the blood without having overt liver disease. The level gradually falls when the individual refrains from alcohol ingestion.

Cholecystitis

Inflammation of the gall bladder (cholecystitis) is often associated with the presence of gallstones. If a gallstone becomes dislodged it can cause inflammation and obstruction of the bile ducts. Symptoms are abdominal pain and fever. Biochemically there are elevated bilirubin and liver enzyme levels. In cholecystitis these parameters are slightly increased but may rise substantially if the bile duct becomes obstructed. The hyperbilirubinaemia is due predominantly to conjugated bilirubin (see *Box 18.3*). *Table 18.2* shows some biochemical changes which would be expected in a number of conditions that lead to hyperbilirubinaemia.

Box 18.3 Gallstones

The most common type of gallstone is made of cholesterol and it is estimated that up to 20% of people on a western diet will develop gallstones in their lifetime. They form in bile supersaturated with cholesterol, which is increased in level relative to phospholipids; normally cholesterol and phospholipid are in a 1:1 ratio. Cholesterol crystallizes out of solution most often in the gall bladder because here the bile is concentrated and often static, giving a greater chance for a crystallization nuclei to initiate lithogenesis (stone formation). The tendency to produce supersaturated or lithogenic bile is inherited and is found more frequently in females than males. There is also an association with obesity.

Pigmented gallstones are less than 25% cholesterol and contain calcium bilirubinate, calcium phosphate and calcium carbonate.

In 1987 a patient at Worthing Hospital had 23 530 gallstones removed after complaining of abdominal pain.

Table 18.2 General changes seen in tests for liver function for different conditions

Condition	Bilirubin	Transaminases	Alkaline phosphatase	Urinary bilirubin
Haemolytic disease	↑↑	N	N	Negative
Hepatitis	↑↑	↑↑↑	↑	Positive
Cholestatic disease	↑↑↑	↑	↑↑↑	Positive

N, normal level.

18.5 INVESTIGATION OF LIVER DISEASE

In the clinical biochemistry laboratory the routine assessment of liver function usually involves measuring the blood levels of total bilirubin, liver enzymes and albumin. If necessary, a number of follow-up tests can be performed, which can give more specific information if a particular disease is suspected. *Table 18.3* shows the common front-line tests performed and a selection of more commonly performed follow-up tests.

Bilirubin

Total bilirubin is usually measured by forming a blue-coloured azobilirubin by reacting bilirubin with alkaline, diazotized, sulphanilic acid; this is known as the **Jendrassik–Grof** method. Only conjugated bilirubin will react and form a blue product in the absence of an accelerator and this is known as direct-reacting bilirubin or **direct bilirubin**. To measure total bilirubin an

Table 18.3 Liver function tests carried out in a clinical biochemistry laboratory

Front-line tests	Follow-up tests
Total bilirubin	Congugated, uncongugated and free bilirubin
Aminotransferases	Bile acids
Alkaline phosphatase	Ammonia
γ-Glutamyltransferase	Bromosulphthalein excretion test
Albumin	Specific proteins, e.g. α_1-antitrypsin, α-foetoprotein, caeruloplasm, coagulation factors
Urinary bilirubin and urobilinogen	

accelerator reagent must be added, which is usually a caffeine–benzoate reagent. In the presence of the accelerator, unconjugated bilirubin also becomes diazotized to form a blue azobilirubin. As unconjugated bilirubin requires an accelerator to react, it is sometimes known as indirect-reacting bilirubin or **indirect bilirubin**.

Rapid measurement of bilirubin in babies is often performed using a direct reading 'bilirubinometer'. A probe which transmits a strong pulse of light from a xenon flash tube is placed on the baby's skin. When triggered, the flash of light illuminates the skin and the bilirubinometer measures how much light is absorbed or reflected (depending on the instrument) by bilirubin, which has an absorbance peak at 454 nm. A direct reading is given of the bilirubin concentration.

Other analytes

Measurement methods of the other front-line analytes involved in the assessment of liver disease are given in other chapters in this book: enzymes are covered in Chapter 10 and measurement details for albumin and other specific proteins are covered in Chapter 12.

Follow-up tests are beyond the scope of this book but the range of tests that are employed testifiy to the fact that the liver is a complicated organ, vital for life. In clinical practice, many different types of technique are used to assess liver function and to aid the diagnosis of liver disease. These range from simple biochemical investigations discussed in this chapter to sophisticated nuclear magnetic resonance scans that can visualize anatomical abnormalities such as tumours. In other types of investigation, biochemical testing of liver enzymes in the cells taken from a liver biopsy can yield information unique to that individual as an asessment for liver transplantation.

SUGGESTED FURTHER READING

In addition to relevant chapters in the text books cited in Chapter 1 the following references are recommended.

Ali S., Friedman S.L. and Mann D.A. (2006) *Liver Diseases: Biochemical Mechanisms and New Therapeutic Insights.* Enfield, NH: Science Publishers.

Burke M.D. (2002) Liver function: test selection and interpretation of results. *Clinics in Laboratory Medicine,* **22**: 377–390.

Ratnavel N. and Ives N.K. (2005) Investigation of prolonged neonatal jaundice. *Current Paediatrics,* **15**: 85–91.

Tredger J.M. and Sherwood R.A. (1997) The liver: new functional, prognostic and diagnostic tests. *Annals of Clinical Biochemistry,* **34**: 121–141.

Westwood A. (1991) The analysis of bilirubin in serum. *Annals of Clinical Biochemistry,* **28**: 119–130.

SELF-ASSESSMENT QUESTIONS

1. What are the important metabolically active cells in the liver?
2. Where does the liver derive its blood supply from?
3. From which compound is bilirubin derived?
4. With which compound is bilirubin conjugated in order to make it water soluble?
5. In the absence of kidney disease, what type of bilirubin can appear in the urine in liver disease?
6. Which type of jaundice would a gallstone cause?
7. What are the two main general categories of liver disease?
8. With which type of liver disease is alkaline phosphatase associated?
9. With which enzyme is alcoholic liver disease associated?
10. Is direct-reacting bilirubin conjugated or unconjugated?

Answers to self-assessment questions

Chapter 1

1. To aid the clinician in diagnosis, screening, monitoring and assessing prognosis by the measurement of biochemical parameters in a patient's sample (usually blood).
2. Imprecision, accuracy, sensitivity and specificity.
3. Inter-individual and intra-individual variation.
4. The range between the values for a given analyte that includes 95% of cases from a reference population, usually a healthy population.
5. The proportion of test results in a disease population that are positive, expressed as a percentage.
6. The proportion of test results in a healthy population that are negative, expressed as a percentage.
7. Anticoagulants.
8. Millimolar (mmol l^{-1}).
9. 0.65 µmol l^{-1}.
10. Temperature, pH and substrate concentration.

Chapter 2

1. Carbohydrate, protein and fat.
2. Vitamins, minerals and trace metals.
3. Marasmus and kwashiorkor.
4. Vitamins A, D, E and K.
5. The concentration should lie between the minimum effective concentration and the minimum toxic concentration.
6. Colorimetry.
7. Colorimetry measures the absorbance at a single wavelength and spectroscopy measures the absorbance of the sample over a range of different wavelengths.
8. 0.5 = 60 700 × 1 × concentration. Concentration = 8.2 µmol l^{-1}.
9. 46.7 mg l^{-1}.

Chapter 3

1. In the stomach.
2. In the cells lining the duodenum.
3. The small intestine.
4. The small intestine.
5. A fall in stomach hydrogen ion concentration.
6. Gastric inhibitory peptide.
7. Stomach, intestine, pancreas and gall bladder.
8. Gastrin.
9. Amylase.
10. Xylose.

Chapter 4

1. Adenine pairs with thymine and guanine pairs with cytosine.
2. A codon.
3. AUG.
4. An exon.
5. It can form a protein that has lost its function.
6. Oncogenes.
7. A tumour suppressor gene or anti-oncogene.
8. Polymerase chain reaction.

Chapter 5

1. Thyroxine, triiodothyronine and calcitonin.
2. A steroid.
3. The free hormone.
4. By binding to a cell surface or an intracellular hormone receptor.
5. The negative feedback loop.
6. The pituitary gland.
7. Hypofunction and hyperfunction.
8. A lowered TSH due to the negative feedback effect of high thyroxine.
9. A stimulation test.
10. A small compound which has only one binding site for antibodies.

Chapter 6

1. Thyroid-binding globulin, pre-albumin and albumin.
2. TRH and TSH.
3. The free hormones.
4. T_3.
5. Primary hyperthyroidism.
6. You would expect high levels of TSH due to the negative feedback.
7. A tumour of the pituitary gland.
8. EMIT.
9. Free T_4 and TSH.

Chapter 7

1. The milliosmole.
2. The kidney.
3. Antidiuretic hormone (AVP) and aldosterone.
4. Stimulates the resorption of sodium ions.
5. Via the renin–angiotensin system.
6. Diabetes insipidus.
7. Aldosterone and cortisol.
8. The red blood cells have a high potassium content that is released into the plasma when they are lysed.
9. Flame photometry and ion-selective electrodes.
10. No.

Chapter 8

1. Protein-bound, complexed with anions and free.
2. PTH and 1,25-DHCC.
3. It acts to raise the calcium concentration.
4. It increases calcium and phosphate uptake in the intestine.
5. 1,25-DHCC.
6. Malignant disease.
7. Parathyroid glands, kidney, bone and the intestine.
8. A defect in the PTH receptor on the cell surface.
9. Dye-binding methods, electrochemical methods and atomic absorption spectrophotometry.

Chapter 9

1. Insulin and glucagon.
2. Muscle and adipose tissue.
3. Polyuria and polydipsia.
4. Insulin-dependent diabetes and non-insulin dependent diabetes.
5. 10 mmol l^{-1}.
6. Hypoglycaemia
7. They should be fasted overnight.

8. The measurement of the level of glycated protein can give information about average glucose levels in the preceeding weeks.
9. A low blood glucose.
10. Glucose oxidase, glucose dehydrogenase, hexokinase and glucose-6-phosphate dehydrogenase.

Chapter 10

1. Cytosolic enzymes.
2. CK-MM, CK-MB and CK-BB.
3. A post-translational modification of the enzyme.
4. Five.
5. Liver and bone.
6. γ-Glutamyltransferase.
7. Creatine kinase.
8. Hepatic disease.
9. Because the rate of the enzyme reaction is independent of substrate concentration.
10. End-point and kinetic determinations.

Chapter 11

1. Phenylalanine hydroxylase.
2. 75%.
3. 25%.
4. To detect an inborn error of metabolism in the absence of any symptoms.
5. Amino acids, organic acids and sugars.
6. From the amniotic fluid taken by amniocentesis.
7. The ΔF508 mutation.
8. Thin-layer chromatography.
9. Homogentisic acid.
10. Accumulation of substrate, decreased concentration of product and increased concentration of alternative metabolites.

Chapter 12

1. Transferrin.
2. The liver.
3. Albumin.
4. Haptoglobin, caeruloplasmin and α_2-macroglobulin.
5. 25 g l^{-1}.
6. PSA.
7. Specific proteins.
8. The isoelectric point (pI).
9. The positive electrode (anode).

Chapter 13

1. Fatty acids, glycerol and cholesterol.
2. Chylomicrons.

3. Apolipoproteins A, C and E.
4. The liver.
5. Type V.
6. Type III.
7. Hypolipidaemia.
8. HDL.
9. Total cholesterol level, cigarette smoking and hypertension.

Chapter 14

1. $pH = \log_{10} [H^+]^{-1}$.
2. Bicarbonate buffer system.
3. The kidney.
4. pCO_2 and $[HCO_3^-]$.
5. A decreased $[HCO_3^-]$.
6. A decreased pCO_2.
7. Hypoventilation resulting in the elevation of pCO_2.
8. Raising the bicarbonate concentration.
9. A compensated respiratory acidosis.
10. The carbon dioxide electrode is a voltammetric technique and the oxygen electrode is an amperometric technique.

Chapter 15

1. IgG, IgM, IgA, IgE and IgD.
2. 10.
3. Plasma cells.
4. IgG.
5. IgG and IgM.
6. Light chains (kappa or lambda).
7. IgM.
8. A paraprotein.
9. Radial immunodiffusion or the Mancini technique.

Chapter 16

1. Classical and alternative.
2. Opsonization.
3. The membrane attack complex.
4. Cytokines.
5. C-reactive protein and serum amyloid A.
6. It binds free haemoglobin.
7. Alpha and beta interferons.
8. Zero.
9. The alternative pathway.

Chapter 17

1. 1,25-Dihydroxycholicalciferol and erythropoietin.
2. At the glomerulus.
3. In the distal tubule.
4. A concentrated urine.
5. 125 ml min^{-1}.
6. Renal tubular acidosis.
7. Less than 150 mg day^{-1}.
8. High molecular weight proteins.
9. Bilirubin.
10. It 'seeds' the precipitation of stone-forming material.

Chapter 18

1. Hepatocytes.
2. The hepatic artery and the portal vein.
3. Haem.
4. Glucuronic acid.
5. Conjugated bilirubin (water soluble).
6. Post-hepatic (obstuctive) jaundice.
7. Hepatocellular and cholestatic.
8. Cholestatic.
9. γ-Glutamyltransferase.
10. Conjugated.

Index

AR-12

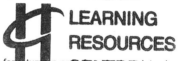

LEARNING
RESOURCES
CENTRE

This book is due for return on or before the last date shown below.

1 7 JAN 2013

1 1 MAR 2013

- 9 DEC 2015

- 9 MAY 2017

WITHDRAWN